Simplex ASD: Data Unravels Phenotypes

Shireen

Table of Contents

Introduction 10

    1.1   book overview 10

    1.2   Background 11

    Epidemiology and genetics of ASD 11

    Phenotypic diversity in ASD 14

    Simplex ASD as a relatively simple model of genetic disease 16

2   Gene dosage changes and phenotype severity in ASD 18

    2.1   Introduction 18

    2.2   Results 21

    Variability in NMD-induced dosage decreases for LGD mutations in different exons 21

    Variability in the sensitivity of phenotypes to changes in the dosage of different genes 30

    Relationships between gene dosage changes and the severity of ASD phenotypes 31

    Inference of quantitative phenotypes based on changes in gene dosage 35

    2.3   Methods 41

    SSC sequencing and phenotype data 41

    VIP sequencing and phenotype data 41

    Phenotype scores analyzed in SSC and VIP 42

    GTEx genotype and expression data 42

Quantification of allele-specific expression (AE).. 43

Gene expression changes due to LGD variants in GTEx 44

BrainSpan expression data.. 52

Dosage-based model of phenotypic effect.. 52

Linear model-based predictions of the effects of LGD mutations....................... 54

3   Autism phenotypes and the exon-intron structure of genes................................ 56

    3.1   Introduction.. 56

    3.2   Results.. 57

Exon-specific phenotypes for *de novo* LGD mutations in ASD........................... 57

Exon-specific gene- and isoform-level dosage changes due to LGD variants 68

Phenotypic consequences of LGD mutations across gene and protein sequences 73

Phenotypic consequences of LGDs affecting functional coding sequences................ 81

    3.3   Methods... 87

Genetic and phenotypic data.. 87

Normalization of phenotypic scores 87

Registration of splice site mutations to exons.. 88

Comparison of phenotype variability.. 88

Chromosomal distance between mutations.. 89

Protein sequence analyses... 89

Distance-matched permutation tests 90

Identifying protein domains affected by LGD mutations 91

Enrichment of mutations in developmentally biased exons 92

Analysis of NMD induced by LGD variants in GTEx 93

Isoform-specific expression changes due to LGD variants 93

4   Properties of exons and genes harboring LGD mutations in ASD 95

    4.1   Introduction 95

    4.2   Results 97

        Developmental expression of exons harboring LGD mutations 97

        Cell type-specific expression biases in ASD-associated genes 99

        Phenotypes associated with expression biases toward neuronal cell types 105

        Combined effects of dosage changes and cell-type specificity 106

    4.3   Methods 111

        Enrichment of mutations in developmentally biased exons 111

        Cell-type specific expression biases 111

        Grouping ASD-associated genes by biological function 112

        Standardization of ASD phenotypes 114

        Calculation of aggregated phenotype scores 114

Conclusion 117

References 120

Introduction

Recent advances in neuropsychiatric genetics [1-4] and, specifically, in the study of autism spectrum disorders (ASD) [5-8] have led to the identification of multiple genes and specific cellular processes that are affected in these diseases [5, 6, 8-10]. However, phenotypes usually associated with ASD vary considerably across autism probands [11-14], and the nature of this phenotypic heterogeneity is not well understood [15, 16]. Despite the complex genetic architecture of ASD [17-22], a subset of cases from simplex families, i.e. families with only a single affected child among siblings, are known to be strongly affected by *de novo* mutations with severe deleterious effects [8, 23, 24]. Interestingly, despite having relatively simpler genetic architecture, simplex autism cohorts often display as much phenotypic heterogeneity as more general cohorts [25-27]. This provides an opportunity for an in-depth exploration of the etiology of the autism phenotypic heterogeneity, at least for these cohorts, using accumulated phenotypic and genetic data. In the presented work, we performed such an investigation of genotype-to-phenotype relationships in ASD.

1.1   book overview

In the presented studies, we investigated the effects of *de novo* LGD mutations on cognitive and other important ASD-related phenotypes, including adaptive behavior, motor skills, communication, and coordination. Initial analyses of LGD mutations both in large-scale sequenced human populations and in two independent simplex ASD cohorts [28, 29] revealed quantitative relationships between changes in gene dosage induced by nonsense-mediated decay (NMD) and the effects of LGD mutations on cognitive and behavioral phenotypes. We then explored simple linear models relating losses of gene dosage to the severity of ASD phenotypes.

To that end, we introduced a genetic parameter, the phenotype dosage sensitivity (PDS), quantifying the change in a specific autism phenotype per unit change in a target gene's dosage. These analyses showed that changes in dosage can explain a significant fraction (~40%) of the variability of autism phenotypes in specific probands. We further investigated whether, due to consistent patterns of exon usage, LGD mutations in the same exon would result in (1) similar dosage changes in the target genes and, consequently, (2) in similar autism phenotypes. We demonstrated that truncating mutations in the same exon often led to similar phenotypes in unrelated ASD probands. We observe consistent patterns of phenotypic heterogeneity for multiple important autism phenotypes and validated these findings in independent ASD cohorts. Finally, we investigated associations between phenotype severity and the developmental expression of exons as well as the expression of ASD-associated genes in neuronal cell types.

1.2   Background

Epidemiology and genetics of ASD

Autism spectrum disorders (ASD) are a group of psychiatric disorders characterized by two core phenotypes: (1) the impairment of social interactions and communication and (2) patterns of repetitive behaviors and restricted interests [30]. The prevalence of ASDs is estimated to be 1 in 59 (~1.5%) [31], with a substantial genetic risk component (estimated heritability ~40-90%) [17, 32, 33]. Notably, ASD presents two distinct patterns of inheritance [17, 34], namely multiplex autism, in which multiple individuals in a family are affected through the transmission of inherited variants, and simplex (or sporadic) autism, in which only a single member of a family is affected.

Recent progress in ASD genetics suggests that diverse genetic insults, including copy number variation [7, 35], rare and *de novo* single nucleotide variants [36], regulatory variants [37], and common inherited polymorphisms [17, 19, 38], contribute to these disorders. Recent large-scale sequencing studies in simplex families have demonstrated strong enrichment of *de novo* mutations among probands. Highly damaging, so-called likely gene-disrupting (LGD) *de novo* mutations (including nonsense, frameshift, and splice-site mutations), in particular, are estimated to contribute to ~30% of simplex cases [8, 39]. Of an estimated 500-1000 ASD risk genes susceptible to LGD mutations, more than 100 genes have been implicated with genome-wide significance [9, 40].

Given the diversity of risk genes targeted by LGD mutations (Figure 0.1), ongoing studies have characterized the functional properties of ASD-associated genes [6, 12, 41], for example in terms of their molecular pathways, positions on biological networks, and spatial and temporal expression patterns. Such studies suggest that important cellular functions – including cytoskeletal and axonal projections, synapse formation, ion channel signaling, chromatin modification [35], and the developmental regulation of transcription – are likely perturbed by mutations in ASD [40, 41]. Notably, investigations of the spatial expression patterns of ASD genes have shown nearly ubiquitous expression throughout the brain [41] (Figure 0.2), and suggest that multiple regions of the brain are likely to be affected [41-43].

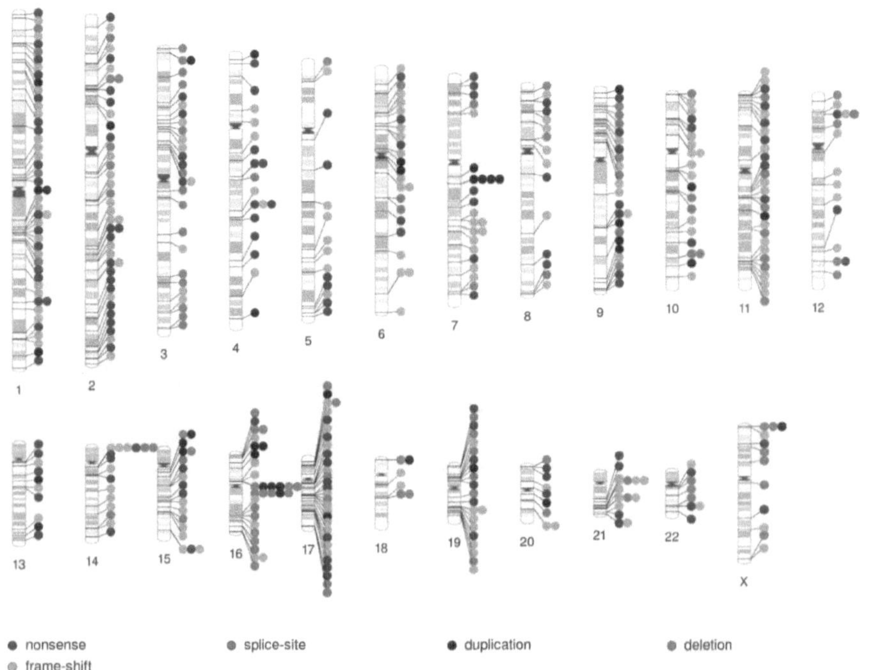

Figure 0.1 Diversity of ASD risk genes affected by *de novo* LGDs and CNVs. Each numbered band represents a human chromosome. Points represent the locations of *de novo* LGD mutations and CNVs observed in simplex ASD populations. Lines between points and chromosomes indicate the chromosomal location of each genetic insult. Colors represent different classes of mutations: nonsense (blue), frameshift (yellow), splice-site (red), and duplication (black) and deletion (purple) CNVs.

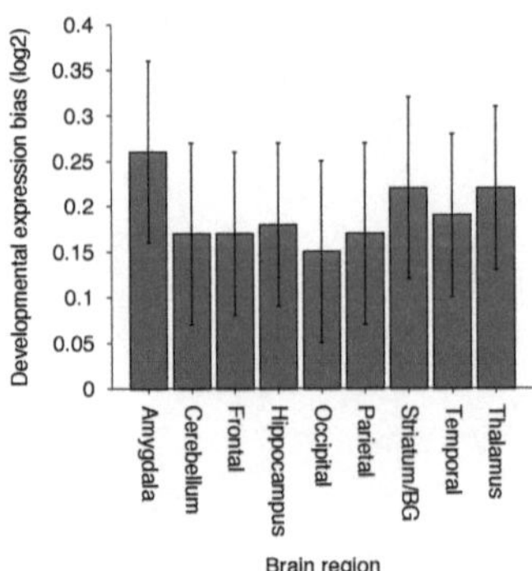

Figure 0.2 Expression bias towards regions of the human brain. Each bar represents the expression bias, calculated as the difference between the median expression levels ASD and control genes, for nine anatomical regions of the human brain. Bars are ordered alphabetically along the x-axis. The y-axis represents the observed expression bias. As the control gene set, we considered genes with nonsynonymous mutations in unaffected siblings in the SSC cohort. Error bars represent SEM estimated by statistical bootstrapping.

These findings constitute important steps towards understanding the cellular and molecular effects of mutations underlying ASD. However, the phenotypic consequences of perturbations to these pathways, for example at the levels of neuronal circuit dynamics [44, 45] and complex cognitive and behavioral phenotypes [26, 46, 47], are not well understood.

Phenotypic diversity in ASD

Connecting genetic insults mechanistically to complex cognitive and behavioral phenotypes remains a key challenge in the study of psychiatric disease. In autism, for example, affected individuals exhibit substantial heterogeneity in both autistic and autism-associated traits. Investigations of the nature of such heterogeneity, however, are challenging due to the relatively complex genetic architecture of ASDs. To wit, many types of genetic insults (i.e. common, rare, and *de novo* variants, both SNVs and CNVs) are likely to contribute; moreover, genetic contributions to the disease, from both rare variants [1, 8, 41] and common polymorphisms [17,

19, 48, 49], are likely to be distributed over many hundreds of genes [50]. How these diverse and distributed genetic insults contribute to disease phenotypes is not well understood.

Several studies have reduced the complexity of such analyses by considering the phenotypes associated with mutations in specific genes [51] or at specific loci [52, 53]. Many studies of monogenic (or syndromic) forms of autism (for example, due to mutations in CHD8 [54], DYRK1A [55, 56], and MECP2 [57, 58]) have identified considerable phenotypic heterogeneity, even within gene-first syndromic cohorts. Similarly, diverse phenotypes are often associated with ASD-associated CNVs at the same locus (for example 16p11.2 [59], 7q11, and 15q11.2-13.3 [60]). Interestingly, ASD cohorts are phenotypically diverse, even when cases are associated with mutations in the same gene.

An alternate approach to studying phenotypes investigates how different types of genetic variation contribute to differences in phenotypes, averaged across many genes. Previous studies have found, for example, that LGD *de novo* mutations are likely to contribute to more severe cognitive [8] and motor skill phenotypes [24]. Other studies further suggest that the severity of ASD-associated behavioral phenotypes reflects contributions from both common and rare variants [22, 61]. These results provide important insights into the overall effects of mutation types. However, even for probands affected by similar types of genetic insults (for example, truncating *de novo* mutations) there remains substantial phenotypic heterogeneity [8, 16, 19, 24, 48]. Importantly, the relationships between specific single variants and observed phenotypes in specific affected individuals (and why variants result in more or less severe phenotypes) are not well understood.

We illustrated these open questions through a simple analysis of proband phenotypes in a well-studied simplex ASD cohort, the Simons Simplex Collection [62]. Specifically, we compared the phenotypes between individuals who were affected by different *de novo* LGD

mutations affecting the same gene. Notably, such probands harbored mutations both of the same

type and truncating the same target gene. The differences in nonverbal IQ observed between

such proband pairs were, at most, ~10% smaller than differences between random probands in

the cohort (Figure 0.3). Moreover, despite the stratification in the analysis by both mutation type

and affected gene, these differences were not statistically significant. Our primary goal in the

following studies was to explore the nature of and mechanisms underlying such phenotypic

differences across individual ASD probands.

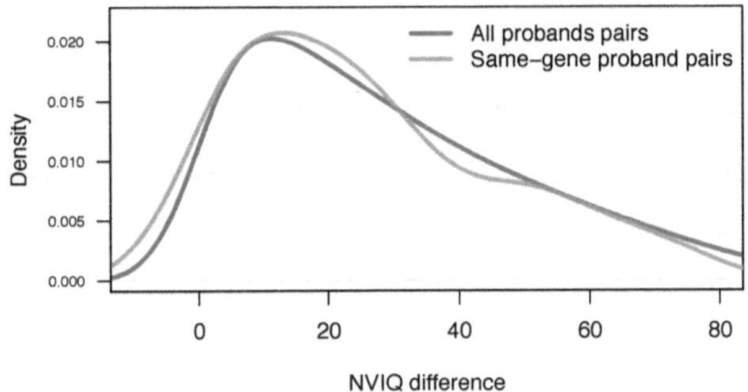

Figure 0.3 Variability of phenotypes for probands with LGD mutations in the same gene. Each
line represents the distribution of pairwise difference in nonverbal IQ (NVIQ) between probands either
paired randomly (grey) or paired by both class of mutation and target gene (i.e. both probands had LGD
de novo mutations affecting the same gene) (red). The x-axis represents the absolute difference in NVIQ
between probands. The y-axis represents the probability density of the distribution.

Simplex ASD as a relatively simple model of genetic disease

In our work, we focused on the contribution of LGD *de novo* mutations to phenotypic

diversity in simplex ASD. Importantly, sporadic simplex cases of ASD and, in particular, probands from quad families (i.e. families with unaffected siblings), are known to be strongly

affected by *de novo* mutations with severe deleterious effects [8, 23, 24, 63]. Given their high

penetrance (~20-40%) and large effect sizes, these mutations are likely to have especially

pronounced (i.e. observable) phenotypic effects. Moreover, because such damaging mutations

are relatively rare (~0.2 per proband), most probands (>95%) affected by an LGD mutation will

harbor no other mutations of comparable effect size (Figure 0.4). Due to their relatively simpler

genetic architecture, the phenotypes resulting from these cases can be attributed to single causal

LGD mutations. Notably, simplex cohorts often display phenotypic heterogeneity comparable to

more general ASD cohorts [8, 26, 27]. Thus, genotype-to-phenotype relationships in autism may

be directly investigated by analyzing the properties of *de novo* LGD mutations and their

associated phenotypes in affected simplex probands.

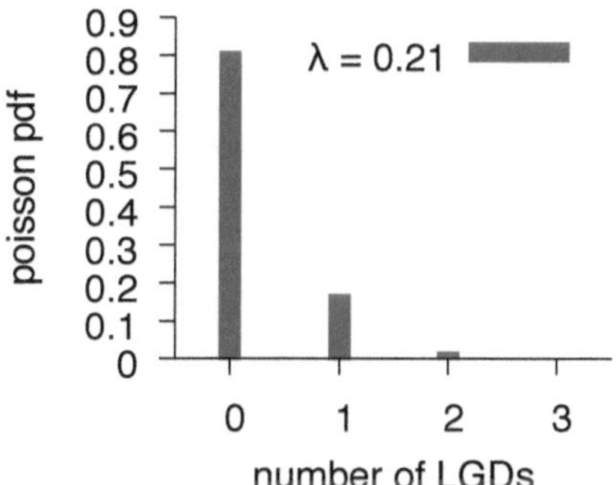

Figure 0.4 Probability of observing different numbers of LGD mutations in a proband. The x-axis represents the number of *de novo* LGD mutations harbored by a proband. The y-axis represents the probability density function, estimated as a Poisson distribution with mean parameter equal to the rate of LGD mutations in SSC.

2　Gene dosage changes and phenotype severity in ASD

2.1　Introduction

Changes in gene dosage, commonly defined as the copy number of a gene, are an important source of genetic variation likely to have large effects on human phenotypes. For example, loss of dosage, such as through copy number or truncating variation, is an important risk factor for many diseases. Recent large-scale genetic studies of psychiatric disorders in general, and of autism spectrum disorders (ASD) specifically, have demonstrated that such genetic insults contribute to the etiology of these diseases. However, even within simplex ASD cohorts, where the effects of such damaging mutations should be least affected by differences in genetic background, probands with truncating mutations in the same genes, i.e. with the same copy number of a target gene, often vary considerably in phenotype (Figure 0.3). The nature of these variations in phenotype is not well understood. In the presented work, we investigated how truncating (nonsense, splice-site, and frameshift) mutations, often called likely gene-disrupting (LGD) mutations, vary in their effects, both on target gene expression and on phenotypes in affected individuals.

Initially we studied how LGD variants differ in their effects on gene expression. Importantly, the mechanisms by which LGDs change expression levels are well-understood, mediated by the highly evolutionarily conserved nonsense-mediated decay (NMD) pathway. Broadly, NMD results in the identification and degradation of mRNA transcripts containing premature truncating codons. However, the effects of NMD on overall expression levels are likely to be affected by both allele-specific expression (AE) and alternative splicing (AS). Both processes have been studied in humans using high-throughput approaches and are known to vary across genes and individuals. Thus, changes in expression due to NMD likely depend on the specifics of AE and AS for the targeted gene in an affected individual. To our knowledge, no prior work analyzed the effects of AE and AS on NMD or modeled their combined effects to quantify changes in total gene expression due to specific LGD variants. In our work, we developed a novel approach to calculate, using RNA-seq data, the extent of NMD in the presence of both AE and AS. We applied our methods to characterize the varying effects of NMD triggered by thousands of LGD variants, in multiple human tissues, and across hundreds of affected individuals.

We then investigated whether gene expression loss due to NMD was a potential mechanism underlying phenotypic variability in ASD. Specifically, we hypothesized that LGD mutations affecting the same gene would vary in their effects on target gene expression, and that the severity of phenotypic consequences resulting from LGDs would be correlated with the magnitude of the changes in expression due to NMD. To that end, we defined gene dosage not as the intact copy number of a gene, as it is commonly used, but as the expression level of an LGD-affected gene relative to its wild-type expression level (i.e. the change in dosage represents the fraction of gene expression lost due to NMD). Using our previously developed methods to analyze NMD as well as genetic and phenotypic data from independent autism cohorts, we investigated how changes in gene dosage affect the severity of cognitive and behavioral phenotypes in autism.

Finally, we explored the quantitative relationships between changes in gene dosage induced by NMD and the phenotypic effects of LGD mutations. To model these relationships, we introduced a genetic parameter, phenotype dosage sensitivity (PDS), characterizing the quantitative relationship between changes in a gene's dosage and changes in specific phenotypes.

Using simple parameterizations, we described how linear models of gene dosage can explain a substantial fraction of the phenotypic heterogeneity in simplex ASD.

2.2   Results

Variability in NMD-induced dosage decreases for LGD mutations in different exons

Initially, we sought to understand how nonsense-mediated decay (NMD) due to truncating variants [64] affects gene dosage. To quantify changes in dosage, which we defined as the fraction of wild-type gene expression lost due to NMD, we developed a statistical model incorporating the effects of allele-specific expression (AE), alternative splicing (AS), and NMD of transcripts (see Methods; Figure 2.1). In our model, we assumed that heterozygous truncating genotypes, such as in probands with LGD mutations observed in ASD, result in transcription from both alleles, possibly in unequal proportions due to regulatory variation (i.e. AE). We further assumed that, due to splicing (AS), only a fraction of transcripts from the affected gene copy would include the exon harboring an LGD variant. Finally, we assumed that NMD is an imperfect process resulting in degradation of a fraction of transcripts susceptible due to incorporation of the LGD variant. In our model we parameterized each of these biological processes using appropriate statistical distributions and then developed an empirical Bayes algorithm to fit the model parameters using RNA-sequencing data (see Methods; Figure 2.2).

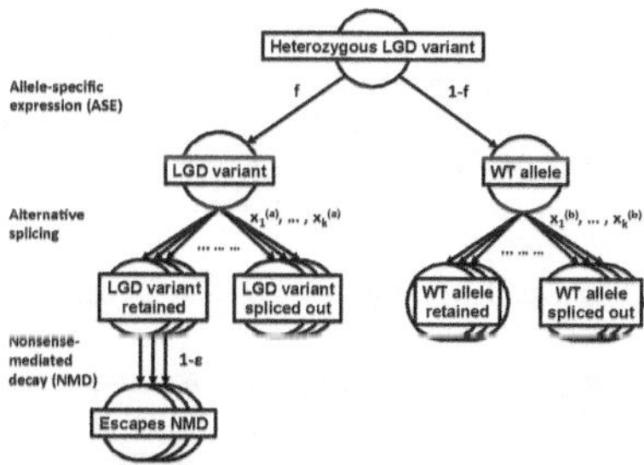

Figure 2.1 Biological processes considered in the modeling of NMD. Each plate represents a gene or transcript sequence. From top to bottom, levels of the diagram represent: (1) the heterozygous genotype of the target gene, (2) transcription of from each of the alleles, (3) alternative splicing into

different isoforms, and (4) reduction in mRNA expression levels due to nonsense-mediated decay (NMD). Arrows between sequences represent the biological processes of allele specific expression (parameterized by *f*), alternative splicing (parameterized by the vector of isoform-specific expression levels, *x*), and NMD (parameterized by the efficiency of degradation, ε). Labels next to each arrow represent the parameters used to model each process in the model (see Methods).

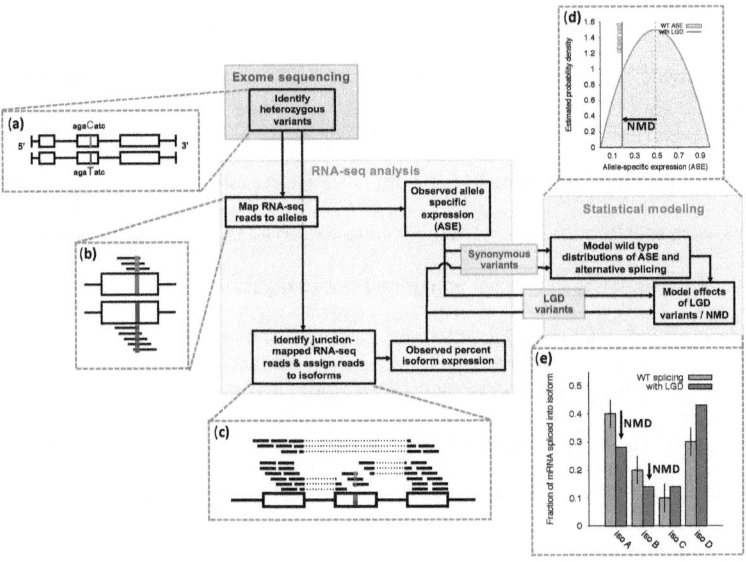

Figure 2.2 Diagram illustrating data analyses used to estimate the effects of NMD. Colored boxes in the flow-chart represent data analyses grouped by the type of data used; counter-clockwise from top, blue represents analysis of sequenced exomes, grey represents the fitting of parameters to RNA-seq data, and beige represents the comparisons between RNA-seq data for synonymous and LGD variants. Inset boxes illustrate calculations used in each analysis: (a) identification of heterozygous genotypes in sequenced exomes, (b) mapping of RNA-seq reads to each allele, (c) quantification of isoform-specific expression, (d) estimation of NMD efficiency from allelic expression, and (e) estimation of NMD efficiency from isoform-specific expression (see Methods).

We applied our model to data from the ongoing Genotype and Tissue Expression (GTEx) Consortium project [65, 66], which collected exome sequencing and corresponding human gene expression data from human donors across multiple tissues. These data allowed us to investigate the effects of NMD on LGD variants present in human populations over thousands of genes and across hundreds of individuals. We applied our empirical Bayes approach to ~4,400 LGD variants in the GTEx dataset. Specifically, we analyzed allele-specific read counts [65] and estimated the effects of NMD by comparing read counts for truncating variants to read counts for synonymous variants (see Methods; Figure 2.2).

When we calculated the effects of NMD in GTEx, we found that truncating variants result on average in relatively mild effects on gene dosage (~15-30% decrease in dosage; Figure 2.3). To quantify the dosage changes, we separately considered two limiting case assumptions. In our upper bound estimate, we assumed that all transcripts incorporating the LGD variant would result either in nonsense-mediated decay or in the translation of non-functional proteins. Under these assumptions, LGD variants resulted in an average dosage change of 31.0% (Figure 2.3, orange line). In our lower bound estimate, we assumed that all transcripts incorporating the LGD variant can be translated into a partial but functional protein. Under these assumptions, where the only loss of dosage was due to NMD, we estimated that LGD variants would cause a 16.4% change in dosage (Figure 2.3, purple line). In both models, we found that heterozygous truncating genotypes resulted in a range of possible dosage changes across approximately three orders of magnitude.

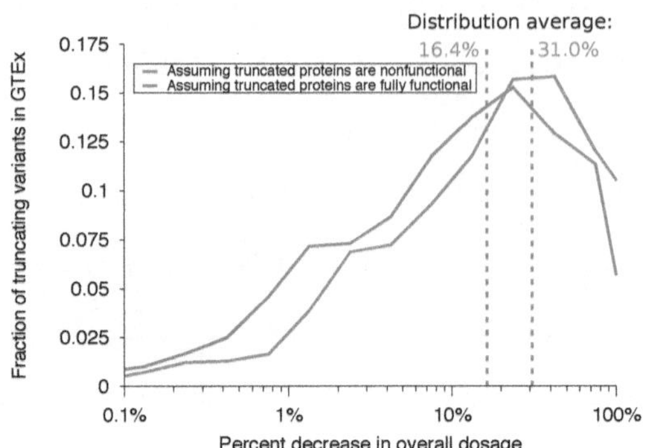

Figure 2.3 The distribution of changes in overall gene expression dosage due to LGD variants in GTEx. For each LGD variant in GTEx, we calculated the relative (percent) change in total gene expression caused by the LGD variant in one of 10 major tissues analyzed in GTEx (see Methods); the results were combined across tissues. Each colored line represents the distribution of estimated dosage changes across all variants. The purple line represents the change in overall gene dosage due to nonsense-mediated decay (NMD) assuming that truncated proteins are fully functional. The distribution in orange represents the change in overall gene dosage assuming that all truncated proteins are nonfunctional. The vertical dashed lines represent the average of each distribution.

We then investigated differences in NMD across tissues. We found that across hundreds of genes, the average NMD efficiency across tissues was similar, with inter-tissue efficiencies of 0.55-0.82 (mean = 0.68; SD = 0.07; CV = SD/mean = 0.097). We also found that the standard deviation of efficiency across variants in a given tissue was inversely correlated with the average efficiency observed in the tissue (Pearson's R = -0.74, $p = 6\times10$-5; Spearman's $\rho = -0.73$, $p =$ 1.4×10^{-4}; Figure 2.4), though NMD in skin (sun exposed) tissue did not seem to follow the trend.

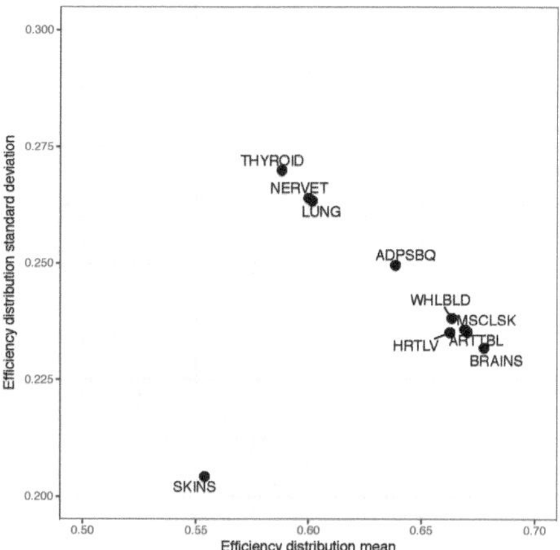

Figure 2.4 Relationship between averages and standard deviations of NMD efficiency in tissues. Each point represents one of ten tissues from GTEx used to estimate the efficiency of NMD. The x-axis represents the average efficiency of NMD observed in the tissue. The y-axis represents the standard deviation of NMD efficiency in the tissue. Statistics for efficiency were calculated across all rare heterozygous LGD variants.

Truncating variants in highly expressed exons should lead, on average, to relatively larger NMD-induced decreases in overall gene dosage. To confirm this hypothesis, we calculated, for each exon harboring a truncating variant, its expression level relative to the expression level of the corresponding gene. We then explored the relationship between the relative expression of exons and the observed NMD-induced decreases in gene expression. The analysis indeed revealed a strong correlation between the relative expression levels of exons harboring LGD variants and the corresponding changes in overall gene dosage (Figure 2.5; Pearson's R = 0.69, p < 2×10^{-16}; Spearman's ρ = 0.81, p < 2×10^{-16}; see Methods).

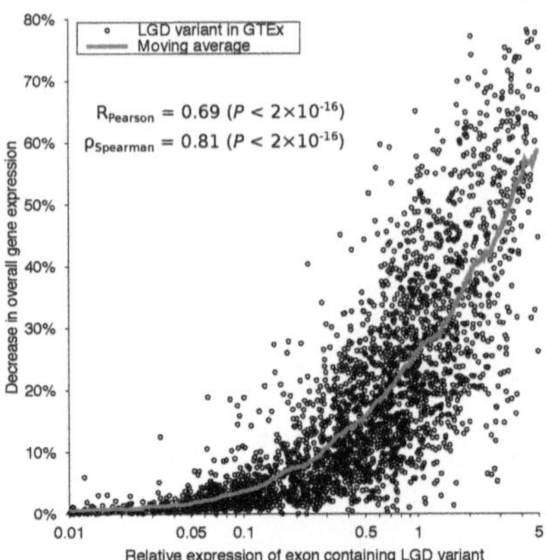

Figure 2.5 Relationship between the relative expression of exons containing LGD variants and the corresponding NMD-induced decreases in overall gene expression. Each point corresponds to the quantification of NMD, in one of ten human tissues, for an LGD variant. The x-axis represents the relative expression of the exon harboring an LGD variant in a tissue; the relative expression of an exon was calculated as the ratio between the exon expression and total expression of the corresponding gene (see Methods). The y-axis represents the NMD-induced decrease in overall gene expression (see Methods). Red line represents a moving average of the data, calculated on an interval of width 0.1 (log-scaled).

To validate our findings, we analyzed data from a CRISPR/Cas9 genetic editing experiment in HAP1 cell lines [67, 68], in which nearly all possible single nucleotide variants (~3,900 SNVs, including 130 LGDs) were introduced into target exons in the BRCA1 gene. Changes in dosage were quantified by calculating the mRNA expression level for cells affected by an LGD mutation relative to the expression levels measured in cells with synonymous mutations. Reassuringly, the observed NMD efficiency in these experiments was similar to the estimates we made using GTEx data (mean = 0.59, SD = 0.24). In addition, we indeed found that the relative expression of target exons (i.e. expression level of the exon divided by expression level of the gene) correlated with changes in dosage due to NMD triggered by LGD mutations in the exon (Pearson's R = 0.65, p = 0.02; Spearman's ρ = 0.61, p = 0.03; Figure 2.6).

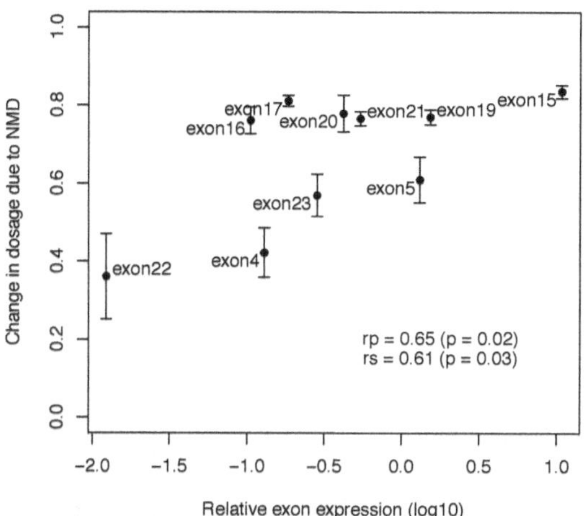

Figure 2.6 Relationship between relative exon expression and change in dosage due to NMD in BRCA1 experiments. Each point represents an exon in BRCA1 targeted for mutagenesis in saturation genetic editing experiments. The x-axis represents the relative expression of the exon, defined as the average expression level of the exon divided by the average expression level of the gene. The y-axis represents the observed change in BRCA1 gene dosage due to LGD mutations in the exon. Error bars represents the SEM.

We then asked whether the *de novo* LGD mutations contributing to ASD would also similarly vary in their effects on target gene expression. To that end, we analyzed *de novo* LGD mutations identified in ~2500 sequenced probands in the Simons Simplex Collection (SSC) [62] When we applied our model of NMD to estimate the dosage changes (i.e. fraction of wild-type expression lost) due to LGD mutations in these datasets, we indeed found that changes in dosage varied substantially across mutations (mean = 0.28; SD = 0.18; CV = SD/mean = 0.65; Figure 2.7). In these calculations, we used the underlying distribution parameters fitted to data from all brain samples in GTEx.

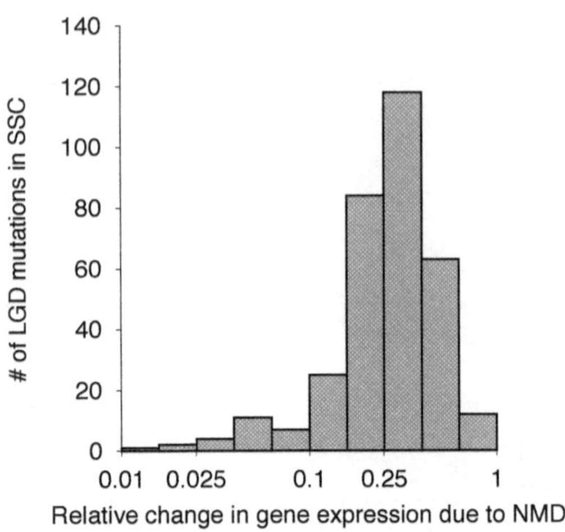

Figure 2.7 Distribution of estimated dosage changes for LGD mutations in SSC. The histogram represents the distribution of the predicted dosage changes resulting from NMD of LGD mutations in SSC. The x-axis (log-scaled), represents the estimated change in dosage. The y-axis represents the number of LGD mutations in SSC. Dosage changes were estimated based on a moving average of dosage changes observed in brain tissues in GTEx (see Methods).

Based on these results, we hypothesized that differences in dosage lost due to NMD of LGD mutations could contribute in part to the phenotypic variability between ASD probands. To investigate, we asked whether larger changes in gene dosage from LGD mutations would lead to more severe disease phenotypes in autism. In the initial analysis, we considered several cognitive phenotypes, full-scale (FSIQ), nonverbal (NVIQ), and verbal (VIQ) intelligence quotients (IQ) [5, 8, 10], available in SSC. These scores are normalized by age and standardized across a broad range of phenotypes [28]. To account for differences in function across genes, we compared only probands with LGD mutations in the same gene. Specifically, for each gene with multiple LGD mutation in SSC, we stratified probands based on whether the LGD mutations affecting them induced higher or lower than average dosage changes, compared to the average for the gene. Probands affected by higher dosage changes indeed had lower IQs than probands with mutations

28

affected by smaller dosage change, differing, on average, by 11.6 full-scale, 13.5 nonverbal, and

9.5 verbal IQ points (Figure 2.8; FSIQ, NVIQ, VIQ Wilcoxon signed-rank one-tail $p = 0.04$,

0.01, 0.1). Moreover, across all probands with mutations in these genes, larger dosage changes

were correlated with the lower absolute IQ phenotype scores (FSIQ, NVIQ, VIQ Pearson's R = -

0.27, -0.31, -0.17; one-tail $p = 0.03$, 0.01, 0.19; Spearman's ρ = -0.19, -0.28, -0.11; one-tail p =

0.12, 0.023, 0.4).

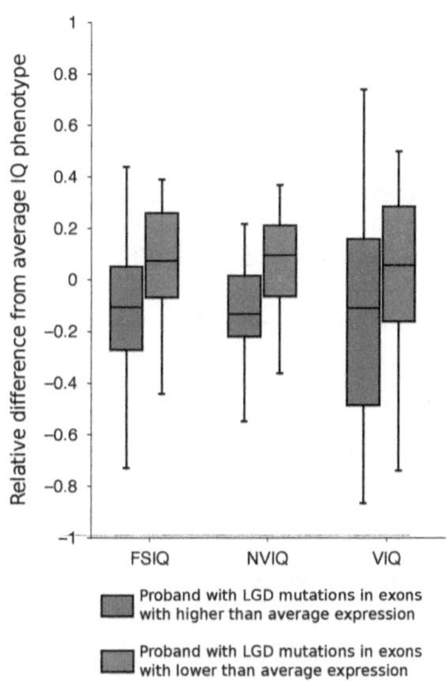

Figure 2.8 IQ phenotypes in probands with LGDs in exons with lower- and higher-than-average expression. Along the x-axis, from left to right, pairs of boxplots are plotted for full-scale (FSIQ), nonverbal (NVIQ), and verbal (VIQ) IQ scores. The y-axis represents the relative IQ score of a proband, defined as the relative deviation of each IQ from the average (i.e. $(x - \mu_x)/\mu_x$). Boxplots show the distribution of relative IQs for probands with LGD mutations in exons with lower-than-average (blue) and higher-than-average (red) expression. The bar in the middle of each box represents the median; the top and bottom of the boxes represent, respectively, the 75th and 25th percentiles. The whiskers represent the minimum and maximum.

We sought to further investigate the relationship between changes in gene dosage and changes in autism phenotypes. It is likely that there is substantial variability across human genes in terms of the sensitivity of intellectual and other ASD phenotypes to gene dosage. Therefore, to quantify the sensitivity of a phenotype, for example IQ, to changes in the expression of specific genes, we considered a simple linear dosage model (see Methods). In the model, we assumed for genes with recurrent truncating mutations in SSC that changes (decreases) in probands' IQs are linearly proportional to the predicted decrease in overall gene dosage due to NMD. We further assumed that each human gene can be characterized by a parameter, which we call its phenotype dosage sensitivity (PDS), characterizing the linear relationship between changes in gene dosage compared to wild type and the corresponding changes in a given human phenotype. Numerically, we defined IQ-associated PDS to be equal to the average change in IQ resulting from a 10% change in gene dosage.

To calculate the sensitivity of IQ phenotypes in autism to changes in dosage, we used the BrainSpan dataset [69], which contains exon-specific expression from human brain tissues. The BrainSpan data allowed us to estimate expression dosage changes resulting from LGD mutations in different exons (see Methods). Using the linear model, for each gene with recurrent truncating ASD mutations, we used predicted changes in gene dosage to estimate gene-specific PDS parameters for intellectual phenotypes (see Methods). Notably, as we expected, PDS values varied substantially across 24 considered human genes (CV = SD/Mean = 0.59, 0.57, 0.72 for FSIQ, NVIQ, VIQ). We restricted this analysis to LGD mutations predicted to cause NMD-induced expression changes, i.e. we excluded mutations within 50 bp of the last exon junction

complex [70], and also assumed the average neurotypical IQ (100) for wild type (intact) gene
dosage.

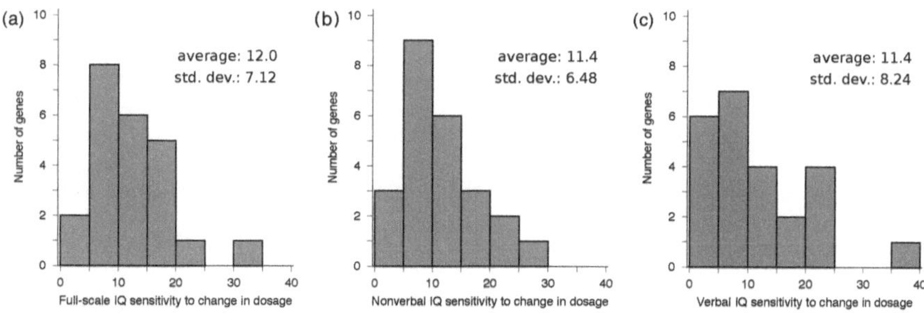

Figure 2.9 Distribution of the sensitivity of IQ phenotypes to changes in gene dosage, i.e. the
Phenotype Dosage Sensitivity (PDS), across different ASD genes with recurrent truncating mutations in
SSC. From left to right, the histograms show the distribution of PDS sensitivity parameters across genes
for (a) full-scale IQ (FSIQ), (b) nonverbal IQ (NVIQ), and (c) verbal IQ (VIQ). To calculate PDS
parameters, we used linear regression, separately for each gene, to fit the relationship between the
observed IQ decrease compared to the neurotypical average value (100) and the estimated change in gene
dosage due to LGD mutations (see Methods). We then calculated PDS as the predicted decrease in IQ due
to 10% decreases in gene dosage.

Relationships between gene dosage changes and the severity of ASD phenotypes

We used the aforementioned linear model to explore the relationship between the relative

expression values of exons (i.e. the ratio of exon expression to gene expression) harboring LGD

mutations and the corresponding decreases in probands' intellectual phenotypes. To account for

differences in phenotypic sensitivity to dosage changes across genes, we normalized the

observed changes in IQ by the estimated PDS values of affected genes. Normalized in this way,

phenotypic effects represent changes in phenotype relative to the predicted effects for 10%

decreases in dosage of affected genes. This analysis revealed that mutation-induced gene dosage

changes are indeed strongly correlated with the normalized phenotypic effects (FSIQ/NVIQ/VIQ

Pearson's R = 0.56, 0.63, 0.51; permutation test p = 0.03, 0.02, 0.02; Figure 2.10). Very weak

31

correlations were obtained for randomly permuted data, i.e. when truncating mutations were randomly re-assigned to different exons in the same gene (average FSIQ/NVIQ/VIQ Pearson's R = 0.11, 0.18, 0.01; SD = 0.23, 0.20, 0.21; see Methods). Since the heritability of intelligence is known to substantially increase with age [71], we also investigated how the results depend on the age of probands. When we restricted our analysis to the older half of probands in SSC (i.e. older than the median age of 8 years), the strength of the correlations between the predicted dosage changes and normalized phenotypic effects increased further (FSIQ/NVIQ/VIQ Pearson's R = 0.68, 0.75, 0.60; permutation test p = 0.03, 0.019, 0.05; Figure 2.11). The strong correlations between target exon expression and intellectual ASD phenotypes suggest that, when gene-specific PDS values are taken into account, a significant fraction (30%-45%) of the relative phenotypic effects of *de novo* LGD mutations across genes can be explained by the resulting dosage changes of target genes.

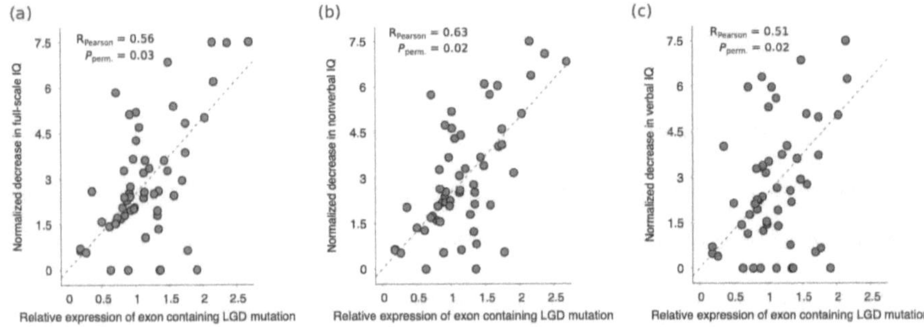

Figure 2.10 Relationship between the relative expression of exons harboring LGD mutations and the corresponding decreases in probands' IQs. From left to right, the scatterplots show (a) full-scale IQ (FSIQ), (b) nonverbal IQ (NVIQ), and (c) verbal IQ (VIQ) scores. Each point in the scatterplots corresponds to a proband in SSC affected by an LGD mutation; only genes with recurrent LGD mutations in SSC were considered. The x-axis represents the relative expression, i.e. the ratio of exon expression to total gene expression, of the exon harboring the LGD mutation. The y-axis represents the proband's observed decrease in IQ (relative to wild-type score of 100) normalized by the Phenotype Dosage Sensitivity (PDS) parameter of each gene (see Methods). Red dashed lines represent the linear regression fits across all points.

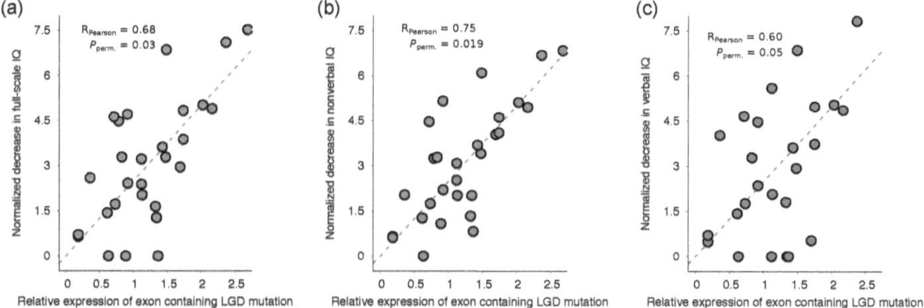

Figure 2.11 Relationship between the relative expression of exons harboring LGD mutations and the corresponding decrease in probands' intellectual phenotypes for the older half of probands in SSC (i.e. older than the median age 8.35 years). From left to right, the scatterplots show (a) full-scale IQ (FSIQ), (b) nonverbal IQ (NVIQ), and (c) verbal IQ (VIQ) scores. Each point in the scatterplots corresponds to a proband in SSC affected by an LGD mutation; only genes with recurrent LGD mutations in SSC were considered. The x-axis represents the relative expression, i.e. the ratio of exon expression to total gene expression, of the exon harboring the LGD mutation. The y-axis represents the proband's observed decrease in IQ (relative to wild-type score of 100) normalized by the Phenotype Dosage Sensitivity (PDS) parameter of each gene (see Methods). Red dashed lines represent the linear regression fits across all points.

We then applied our linear model to study the effects of dosage changes on another quantitative phenotype, adaptive behavior. In SSC and the independent Simons Variation in Individuals project (VIP) [29], behavioral adaptability was scored using the Vineland Adaptive Behavior Scales (VABS) [72], which contained overall composite scores as well as subscores for communication, daily living skills (DLS), and socialization. When we applied the linear dosage model while accounting for the sensitivity of VABS phenotypes to changes in the dosage of different genes (i.e. gene-specific PDS values), we found that normalized VABS phenotypes also correlated with the relative expression of exons harboring LGD mutations. (Pearson's R = 0.75, permutation test p = 0.003; Figure 2.12). Results were consistent in the independent SSC and VIP datasets (in SSC, for example, Pearson's R = 0.73, permutation test p = 0.013). Notably, IQ and VABS scores were only weakly correlated (for NVIQ and VABS composite scores,

Pearson's R = 0.46, $p = 1.50 \times 10^{-4}$).

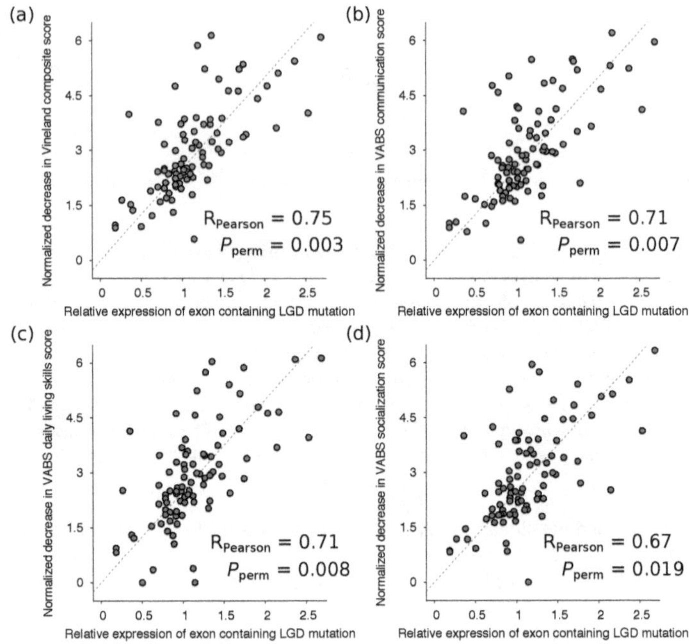

Figure 2.12 Relationship between the relative expression of exons harboring LGD mutations and the corresponding decrease in probands' adaptive behavior phenotypes, i.e. Vineland Adaptive Behavior Scales (VABS) in SSC and VIP probands. From top left, the scatterplots show standardized VABS (a) composite, (b) communication, (c) daily living skills, and (d) socialization scores. Each point in the scatterplots corresponds to a proband in SSC or VIP affected by an LGD mutation; only genes with recurrent LGD mutations across both datasets were considered. The x-axis represents the relative expression, i.e. the ratio of exon expression to total gene expression, of the exon harboring the LGD mutation. The y-axis represents the proband's observed decrease in VABS score (relative to wild-type score of 100) normalized by the Phenotype Dosage Sensitivity (PDS) parameter of each gene (see Methods). Red dashed lines represent the linear regression lines across all points.

Using the developmental expression data available in BrainSpan, we then asked whether

changes in dosage at specific developmental periods would correlate more strongly with the resulting proband phenotypes. To that end, we performed the linear model analysis, i.e.

normalizing for the sensitivity of phenotypes to each gene, using relative exon expression data

from each of six developmental periods: early, mid, and late prenatal stages, infancy/childhood,

adolescence, and adulthood. In our analysis, we did not find significant differences between

relative expression levels at different developmental periods (Figure 2.13).

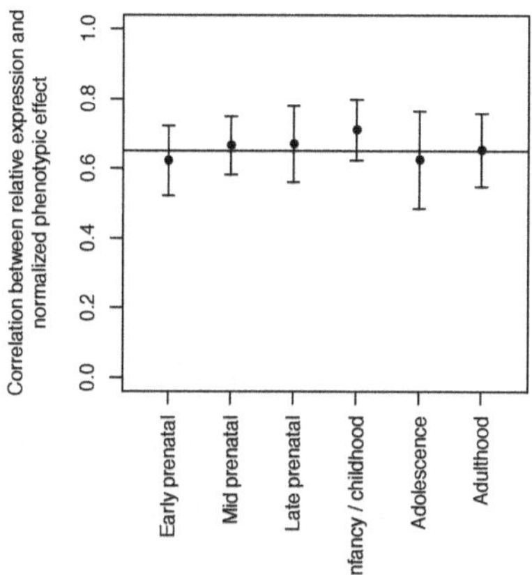

Figure 2.13 Correlation between relative exon expression and normalized phenotypic effects across development. From left to right, the x-axis represents different developmental periods arranged in temporal order. The y-axis represents the correlation between relative expression and normalized phenotypic effects on nonverbal IQ. Relative expression was calculated as mean exon expression level divided by the mean gene expression level in each developmental period. Correlations were calculated using the linear dosage/PDS model (see Methods). Error bars represent standard deviations estimated by statistical bootstrapping.

Inference of quantitative phenotypes based on changes in gene dosage

We then evaluated the ability of our linear dosage model, based on calculated PDS

parameters, to explain the effects of LGD mutations on non-normalized IQ scores. To that end, for each gene with multiple truncating mutations in different probands, we used our linear regression model to perform leave-one-out predictions for IQ scores, i.e. we used PDS values calculated based on all but one probands with mutations in the gene to estimate IQ values for the left out proband (Figure 2.14, inset; see Methods). Despite the simplicity of our model, for LGD mutations that trigger NMD, the model predictions (Figure 2.14, Figure 2.15) were significantly smaller than the median differences between probands with LGD mutations in the same gene (median prediction errors for FSIQ/NVIQ/VIQ were 12.2, 11.0, 20.6 points; same gene median IQ difference 24.0, 22.0, 30.5 points; MWU one-tail test $p = 0.019, 0.014, 0.017$). The inferences based on probands of the same gender (Figure 2.14, Figure 2.15) had significantly smaller errors compared to inferences based on probands of the opposite gender (same gender FSIQ/NVIQ/VIQ median error 11.1, 9.1, 15.9 points; different gender median error 19.0, 19.9, 33.0 points; MWU one-tail test $p = 0.03, 0.018, 0.02$). Moreover, as expected based on our previous analyses, prediction errors decreased for older probands; for example, for probands older than 12 years, median FSIQ/NVIQ/VIQ error 7.0, 7.6, 10.0 points (Figure 2.14, Figure 2.15, Figure 2.16).

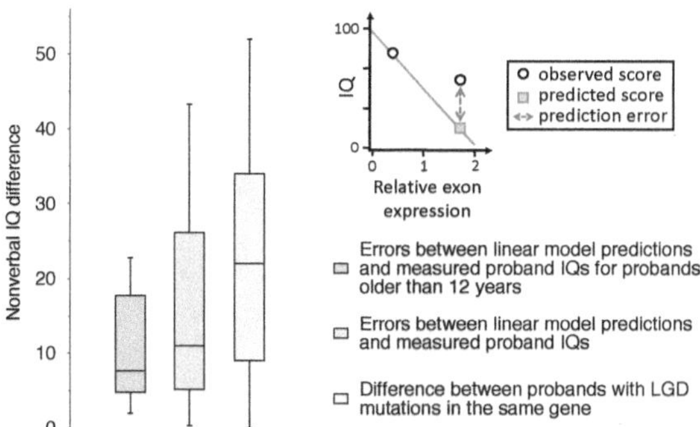

Figure 2.14 Boxplots represent the distribution of errors in predicting the effects of LGD mutations on NVIQ (see Methods); NVIQ prediction errors are shown for all probands (green), and for probands older than 12 years (purple). For comparison, the average differences in NVIQ scores between probands with LGD mutations in the same gene are also shown (blue). Only genes with multiple LGD mutations in SSC were considered. The ends of each solid box represent the upper and lower quartiles; the horizontal lines inside each box represent the medians; and the whiskers represent the 5th and 95th percentiles. The inset panel illustrates the linear regression model used to perform leave-one-out predictions of probands' NVIQs. Round open points represent observed phenotypic scores for probands with LGD mutations in the same gene, the grey square point represents the predicted phenotypic score, and the red dotted line represents the prediction error.

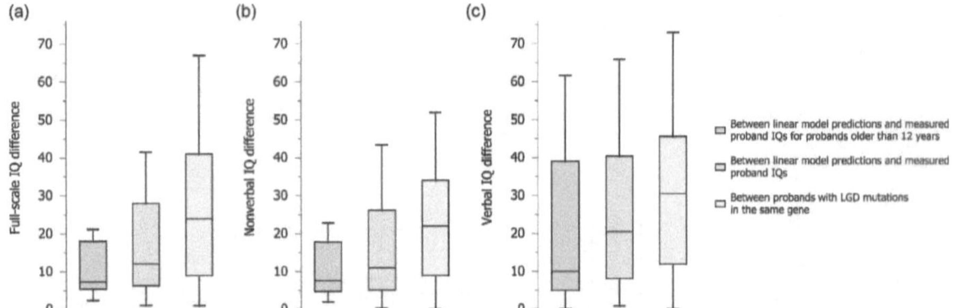

Figure 2.15 Distribution of the errors in predicting the effect of LGD mutations on IQ scores based on the linear dosage model. The errors are shown for all probands (green), and for probands older than 12 years (purple); for comparison, the distribution of IQ differences between all probands with LGD mutations in the same genes are also shown (blue). From left to right, plots represent the distribution of score differences for (a) full-scale IQ (FSIQ), (b) nonverbal IQ (NVIQ), and (c) verbal IQ (VIQ). The ends of each solid box represent the upper and lower quartiles, the horizontal lines within each box represent the medians, and the whiskers represent the 5th and 95th percentiles.

38

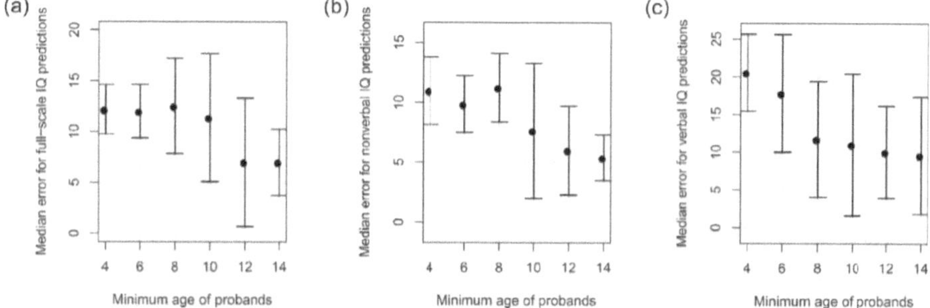

Figure 2.16 Median error in predicting the effects of LGD mutations on IQs for older probands in SSC. From left to right, plots represent the median prediction errors for (a) full-scale IQ (FSIQ), (b) nonverbal IQ (NVIQ), and (c) verbal IQ (VIQ). The x-axis represents the minimum age of probands used for leave-one-out predictions. The y-axis represents the median prediction error based on the linear dosage model. Error bars were estimated using bootstrapping.

Interestingly, we observed in these analyses that the inference errors differed across probands with relatively lower and higher IQ scores. For example, we observed smaller inference errors for probands with IQ >70 compared to ASD probands with IQ ≤70 (for IQ >70 median NVIQ error = 11.0, for IQ ≤70 median error = 16.4; Mann-Whitney U one-tail test p = 0.08). To further explore these differences between the lower and higher IQ probands, we investigated whether using the relative expression of exons during different developmental periods would result in more accurate phenotypic predictions in each cohort. Given the substantial differences in predictions error, we separately investigated phenotypic predictions for the lower IQ (≤70) and higher IQ (>70) probands. Interestingly, we found (Figure 2.17a) that using relative exon expression in early- and mid-prenatal developmental periods resulted in significantly more accurate (by ~35%) phenotypic predictions specifically for lower IQ probands. In contrast, for higher IQ probands we observed (Figure 2.17b) similar accuracy of phenotypic predictions based on exon expression data from different developmental periods.

This result suggests that expression of prenatally biased exons is significantly more informative for phenotypes of the lower IQ cohort.

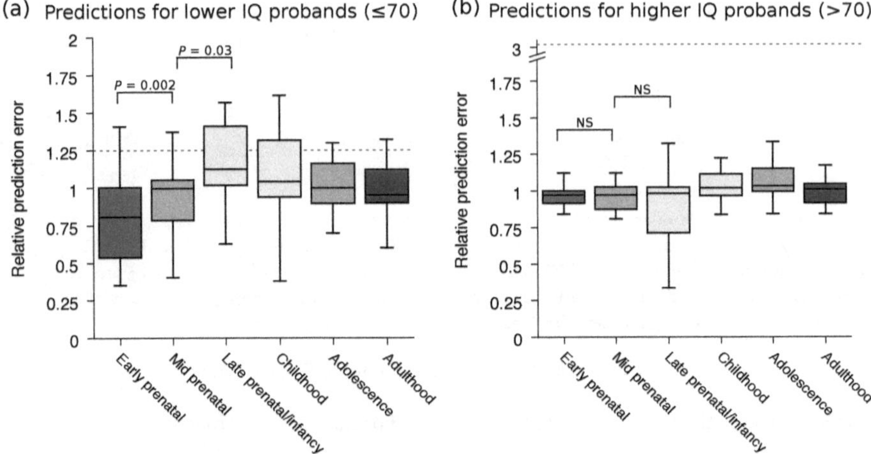

Figure 2.17 Prediction errors using relative expression measured during different developmental periods. For each of six broad developmental periods, we calculated the relative expression of exons targeted by LGD mutations in SSC. We used development-specific relative expression to make leave-one-out predictions of IQ for probands affected by each mutation (see Methods). Boxplots represent the prediction errors for (a) lower IQ probands (nonverbal IQ ≤ 70) and (b) higher IQ probands (nonverbal IQ > 70). The x-axis represents the six developmental periods for which predictions were made. The y-axis represents the relative error of predictions, normalized to the average error across all periods. Horizontal dotted lines indicate the expected median error for predictions based on mutations in the same gene.

2.3 Methods

SSC sequencing and phenotype data

We used exome sequencing and ASD probands' phenotypic data available in the Simons

Simplex Collection (SSC) [28]. *De novo* LGD mutations were obtained from Iossifov *et al.* [8].

As a source of phenotypic data, we used the Prepared Phenotype Dataset (v15) from the SFARI

Base online data portal (sfari.org/resources/sfari-base). The SSC inclusion/exclusion criteria,

phenotype profiling instruments, and sequencing protocols have been described in previous

publications [20, 28, 36, 73, 74].

To identify the effects of mutations on gene transcripts, we analyzed variants in SSC

using Ensembl's Variant Effect Predictor (VEP) tool, which provides multiple annotations for

each mutation based on its predicted effects on different transcriptional isoforms of a gene

(grch37.ensembl.org/info/docs/tools/vep) [75]. For each mutation in SSC, we used VEP to

identify likely gene-disrupting (LGD) mutations by searching for the following predicted

consequences: nonsense (translational stop gained) variants, frameshift indels, splice acceptor

variants, and splice donor variants.

VIP sequencing and phenotype data

We used sequencing and phenotypic data available in the Simons Variation in Individuals

Project (VIP) [29]. *De novo* LGD mutations and the corresponding phenotype scores for affected

probands were obtained from the Simons VIP Phase 2 Single Gene Dataset v4.0, available from

SFARI Base online data portal (sfari.org/resources/sfari-base).

Both SSC and VIP include ASD probands of both genders spanning a broad range of ages and phenotypic abilities. In our analyses, we considered IQ scores (available for SSC only) and Vineland Adaptive Behavior Scales scores (available for both SSC and VIP). Both are normalized to account for developmental differences and hence were suitable for direct comparison between probands.

To investigate the dosage effects across human tissues resulting from protein-truncating variants, we used data from the Genotype-Tissue Expression (GTEx) project [76]. Processed RNA-seq data, including expression data summarized to genes, isoforms, and exons, were obtained through the consortium's online data portal (https://www.gtexportal.org/). Raw sequencing and genotype data were obtained via NCBI's Database of Genotypes and Phenotypes (dbGaP) (Study Accession: phs000424.v6.p1), available online (ncbi.nlm.nih.gov/gap). For RNA-seq data, we obtained SRA submitted files; these files contained the binary alignment map (BAM) for each RNA-seq experiment. In the analysis, we considered samples from ten major human tissues: adipose (subcutaneous), tibial artery, brain, heart (left ventricle), lung, skeletal muscle, tibial nerve, skin (not sun-exposed), thyroid, and whole blood.

In the downloaded genotype data, we identified small indels ($\leq$ 6 bp) and single-nucleotide variants that were called using exome sequencing of 180 individuals (v6 from June 2014). Sequencing and variant calling protocols were previously described in Melé *et al.* [77]. To explore the dosage effects resulting from heterozygous variants, we included only heterozygous genotypes in our analysis. To limit the number of false positive genotypes, we only used calls with quality ≥ 20 (Phred-scale) for SNVs, and ≥ 30 for indels. In addition, to minimize the potential for downstream mapping and short read alignment biases, we excluded SNVs with non-unique flanking regions, based on UCSC mappability tracks. For SNVs, we excluded variants with 50 bp mappability less than one. For indels, we excluded variants with 36 bp mappability less than one. We limited our study to autosomal and rare variants (defined as allele frequency ≤ 0.05).

Quantification of allele-specific expression (AE)

AE for GTEx variants was quantified using RNA-seq data. In general, we followed previously developed protocols based on re-alignment of reads to local sequences containing either wild-type (WT) or variant alleles (tllab.org/data-software) [65]. For each individual, we first identified heterozygous genotypes and then extracted the flanking (± 100 bp) reference genome sequences around each variant to produce a set of local sequences containing WT alleles. Next, we substituted the variant allele into each sequence to reflect the genotyped truncating variant, producing a matching set of local sequences with variant alleles. Short reads from RNA-seq experiments from an individual were then realigned separately against the reference and alternate sequences. To quantify the expression of each allele, we counted the number of reads aligning uniquely and without error to the WT and variant sequences, respectively. These numbers were then used as allele counts reflecting AE.

To extract flanking reference sequences, we used the fastaFromBed tool from the bedtools software suite (v.2.23.0) [78]. All reference sequences were taken from the human reference genome (hg19) provided by GTEx (gtexportal.org). For aligning short reads, we used BWA (v.0.7.3) [79], and kept only alignment calls with base quality ≥ 10 and mapping quality $\geq$

35. Following the methods in Rivas *et al.* [65], we restricted our analysis to samples with at least 8 mapped reads, and to variants with median allele frequency, across all tissues, ≤ 0.95 and ≥ 0.05.

Gene expression changes due to LGD variants in GTEx

To quantify altered gene expression due to an LGD variant, we considered the changes in expression (Δx) compared to wild type as a combined effect of allele-specific expression (AE), alternative splicing (AS), and nonsense-mediated decay (NMD). To account for AE, we reasoned that only a fraction of total mRNA would be transcribed from each allele. To account for alternative splicing, we reasoned that transcripts would be spliced into multiple transcript isoforms, only some of which would retain the exon with the truncating mutation. Finally, we assumed that nonsense-mediated decay is an imperfect degradation process, in which some fraction of LGD-containing mRNA escapes NMD. Formally, we represented a change in expression as:

$$\Delta x = f \cdot \epsilon \cdot x_{\text{exon}} \quad (1)$$

where the parameter f (ranging from 0 to 1) quantifies the fraction of total transcription from the allele harboring the LGD variant, the parameter ϵ (ranging from 0 to 1) quantifies NMD efficiency, and x_{exon} represents the wild-type expression level of transcripts with the LGD-containing exon, i.e. transcripts susceptible to NMD.

Because post-NMD expression levels are experimentally observed, the relationship between measured and wild-type expression levels can be expressed as:

$$x'_{\text{exon}} = x_{\text{exon}} - \Delta x \quad (2)$$

where x'_{exon} represents the experimentally observed expression. Combining equations (1) and (2), we can express the effects of NMD in terms of x'_{exon}:

$$\Delta x = \frac{f \cdot \epsilon}{1 - f \cdot \epsilon} \cdot x'_{\text{exon}} \qquad (3)$$

In order to estimate Δx for each gene, we needed to infer the parameters f and ϵ, which quantify AE and NMD efficiency respectively. As we describe in the following sections, we inferred these parameters probabilistically by fitting appropriate distributions. Notably, because we were interested in comparing the effects of NMD across different tissues, and since the efficiency of NMD may vary across tissues, we performed separate analyses for each tissue.

Parametric inference of AE

To model the expected distribution of f for each gene, we considered the AE observed for rare synonymous variants in the gene because such variants are unaffected by NMD. We considered a hierarchical model in which the distribution of f can be modeled as a beta distribution ($f \sim \text{Beta}(\alpha_f, \beta_f)$), with hyperparameters α_f and β_f. In the model, each specific measurement of a synonymous variant's AE represents a binomial sample with parameter f drawn from the beta distribution: $k \sim \text{Binomial}(n, f)$, where n is the total number of reads from both copies of the gene, and k is the total number of reads from the synonymous variant allele. In this formulation, the inference of the underlying parameters can be performed by fitting a standard hierarchical beta-binomial model [80, 81]. To model the distribution of f in a given gene, we used the maximum *a posteriori* estimators for the beta distribution:

$$\hat{\alpha}_f, \hat{\beta}_f = \underset{\alpha_f, \beta_f}{\text{argmax}} \prod_{v \in V_{\text{syn}}} \prod_{i \in C_v} \left[\int_0^1 P(k_{v,i} \mid n_{v,i}, f) \cdot P(f \mid \alpha_f, \beta_f) \cdot df \right] \cdot P(\alpha_f, \beta_f) \qquad (4)$$

Here, v indexes a specific synonymous variant from the set of all such variants $V_{\text{syn.}}$, and i

indexes a specific individual carrying the variant allele, where C_v is the set of all carriers. $k_{v,i}$

and $n_{v,i}$ are, respectively, the number of reads mapped to the synonymous allele v and the total

number of reads mapped in an AE experiment.

To perform the maximization in equation (4), we used a standard re-parameterization of

$\left(\alpha_f, \beta_f \right)$ into $u = \frac{\alpha_f}{\alpha_f + \beta_f}$ and $v = \frac{1}{\sqrt{\alpha_f + \beta_f}}$ [82]. The parameters (u, v) represent the mean and

approximate standard deviation of the Beta distribution. To find values that maximize the

posterior probability, we divided the parameter space into a discrete grid and used a grid search

algorithm. For the hyperprior distributions, we chose a uniform distribution for the mean and a

commonly used half-Cauchy distribution for the variance [83].

Note that the resulting estimators are based on multiple synonymous variants, each of

which can have multiple individual carriers in the study population. Importantly, we only

considered individuals with matched common synonymous variant alleles in the gene. As a

result, the variance of the fitted distributions accounts for differences across both haplotypes and

individuals. To minimize undersampling effects, we limited our analysis to genes with at least

four different synonymous mutations and at least ten individual carriers.

To infer NMD efficiency (ϵ), we compared the observed AE for LGD variants in GTEx

to the expected AE estimated based on synonymous variants in the affected genes. The relative

difference between the observed and expected values was then used to quantify the efficiency of

NMD. Since experimental measurements for LGD variants are relatively sparse (on average, one experiment per carrier of each LGD variant), we used an empirical Bayes approach to fit a hierarchical model. Specifically, we first used the observed AE for all LGD variants to infer the distribution of NMD efficiency across variants, and then we estimated the likely efficiency of NMD for specific variants.

We assumed that NMD would function with some efficiency $\epsilon \in [0,1]$, and modeled the distribution of ϵ using a Beta distribution ($\epsilon \sim \mathrm{Beta}(\alpha_e, \beta_e)$). In this model, each AE measurement for an LGD variant v corresponds to a binomial sample ($k \sim \mathrm{Binomial}(n, p)$), where k is the number of reads with the LGD variant, n is the total number of reads, and $p(f, \epsilon)$ is the underlying sampling parameter which depends on the AE parameter f of the LGD allele and the NMD efficiency ϵ. $p(f, \epsilon)$ can be expressed as:

$$p(f, \epsilon) = \frac{f \cdot (1 - \epsilon)}{(1 - f) + f \cdot (1 - \epsilon)} = \frac{f \cdot (1 - \epsilon)}{1 - f \cdot \epsilon} \tag{5}$$

Where the numerator expresses the amount of post-NMD mRNA containing the LGD allele, and the denominator expresses the total amount of post-NMD mRNA from both alleles.

To learn the distribution of ϵ across variants, we searched for parameter values that would maximize the posterior probability given all experimental observations. Formally, the maximization can be written:

$$\hat{\alpha}_e, \hat{\beta}_e = \operatorname*{argmax}_{\alpha_e, \beta_e} \prod_{v \in V_{\mathrm{LGD}}} \left[\iint_{f, \epsilon} P_v\big(k \mid n, p(f, \epsilon)\big) \cdot P_v\big(f \mid \hat{\alpha}_f, \hat{\beta}_f\big) \cdot P\big(\epsilon \mid \alpha_e, \beta_e\big) \cdot df \cdot d\epsilon \right] \cdot P(\alpha_e, \beta_e)$$

$$\tag{6}$$

Here, v indexes a specific LGD variant drawn from the set of all analyzed LGD variants (V_{LGD}). The term $P_v\big(k \mid n, p(f, \epsilon)\big)$ represents the likelihood to observe AE for an LGD variant v. However, since $p(f, \epsilon)$, the binomial rate parameter, depends on ϵ and f (see Eqn. 5), the calculation of each likelihood requires integration across both parameters. Overall, the procedure searches for a distribution for ϵ that best explains deviations of AE for LGD variants from the expected AE distribution for each affected gene. The distribution of ϵ gives the likely percent decrease in expression due to NMD.

To perform the optimization, we re-parameterized the beta distribution using mean and variance parameters $u = \frac{\alpha_e}{\alpha_e + \beta_e}$ and $v = \frac{1}{\sqrt{\alpha_e + \beta_e}}$. Then we divided the parameter space into a discrete grid and calculated the posterior probability at each value of (u, v). For the hyperprior distributions, we chose a uniform distribution for the mean and a half-Cauchy distribution for the variance parameter. We calculated the double integrals in Equation (6) numerically using Newton-Cotes cubature.

Using the maximum *a posteriori* values for parameters (α_e, β_e), we then inferred estimates of NMD efficiency for individual LGD variants. For each variant, we searched for maximum *a posteriori* estimates of specific values of ϵ:

$$\hat{\epsilon} \;=\; \underset{\epsilon}{\mathrm{argmax}}\, P\big(k \mid n, p(\epsilon) \big) \cdot P\big(\epsilon \mid \hat{\alpha}_e, \hat{\beta}_e \big) \tag{7}$$

$$\;=\; \underset{\epsilon}{\mathrm{argmax}} \left[\int_0^1 P\big(k \mid n, p(f, \epsilon) \big) \cdot P\big(f \mid \hat{\alpha}_f, \hat{\beta}_f \big) \cdot df \right] \cdot P\big(\epsilon \mid \hat{\alpha}_e, \hat{\beta}_e \big) \tag{8}$$

The prior term was calculated directly from the parameters $\hat{\alpha}_e$ and $\hat{\beta}_e$. To calculate the total likelihood of (k, n), which depends on rate parameter p, we integrated over possible values of f. The maximization in Equation (8), performed for each LGD variant separately, estimates the efficiency of NMD for a specific observed variant.

In our implementation, we estimated values of $\hat{\epsilon}$ using a one-dimensional parameter-scanning algorithm. For each value of ϵ, we evaluated the integral over f numerically, using Simpson's rule quadrature.

Statistical inference of the parameters f and ϵ, described in the previous sections, allowed us to compute the changes in expression due to each LGD variant (see Eqn. 1). To account for differences in absolute expression level across genes, we normalized the effects of NMD by the total expression of affected genes:

$$\Delta x_{\text{rel}} = \frac{\Delta x}{x_{\text{gene}}} = \frac{\Delta x}{x'_{\text{gene}} + \Delta x} \quad (9)$$

Where x_{gene} is the total amount of mRNA expressed and x'_{gene} is the experimentally measured mRNA expression. In this way, Δx_{rel} expresses the normalized (fraction) change in target gene expression due to NMD. In our analyses, we compared Δx_{rel} to the relative expression of exons, defined as the expression level of the target exon divided by the total expression level of the gene.

To evaluate our model, we generated synthetic read counts by simulating the RNA sequencing of variants in genes. We used simulated synonymous variants (i.e. AE datasets) to evaluate our statistical model's ability to recover parameters α_f and β_f for allele-specific expression. We then used simulated LGD variants (i.e. NMD datasets), including the loss of alternative-allele reads due to NMD, to evaluate our model's ability to fit parameter ϵ for specific variants.

For each synthetic AE dataset, we simulated the allele-specific expression of the gene by randomizing parameters for α_f and β_f to generate an underlying distribution for the parameter f. We sampled from the distribution to generate specific values of f in an individual. Then, for each individual, we performed a random binomial sample to generate a specific observation of

reads. The number of reads in each binomial sample was randomly chosen from a Poisson

distribution to match the minimum number of reads in each observation in our experimental

dataset ($\lambda = 8$).

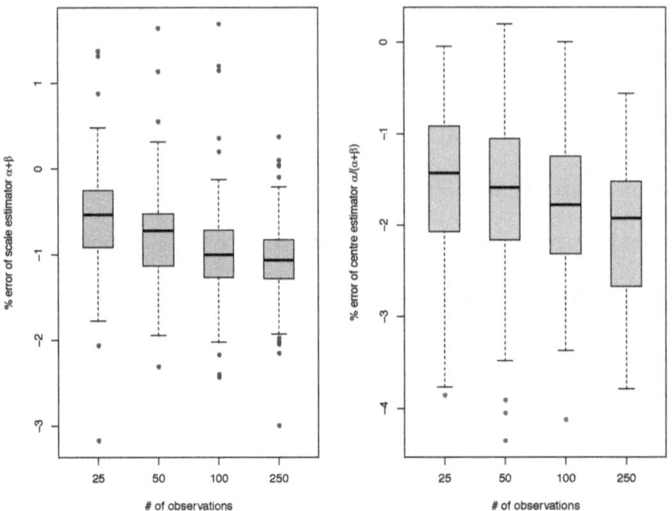

Figure 2.18 Estimation errors for the distribution of allele-specific expression for different
dataset sizes. In each plot, the x-axes represent the number of observations in each synthetic dataset. The
y-axes represent the ($\log_{10}$-scaled) estimation errors for the scale (left) and center (right) parameters of the
AE distribution. Each boxplot represents a distribution of errors observed across 1000 synthetic datasets.
The bars inside of each box represent the median; the top and bottom of each box represent the 25th and
75th percentiles; the whiskers represent the upper and lower bounds of the 95% confidence interval;
points represent outliers.

We then applied our model of AE (see Eqn. 4) to calculate the underlying distribution of

f for each gene in our synthetic dataset. To evaluate the accuracy of the inference, we calculated

the percent error in the resulting (fitted) estimates relative to the initially generated values.

Importantly, these datasets simulate both variability across individuals and sparsity in the number of sequenced reads. Across a randomly generated pool of 10,000 simulated genes, we observed ~3% error in the estimation of the mean, and ~10% error in the estimation of the scale parameter (Figure 2.18). As expected, these errors were inversely proportional to the number of observations.

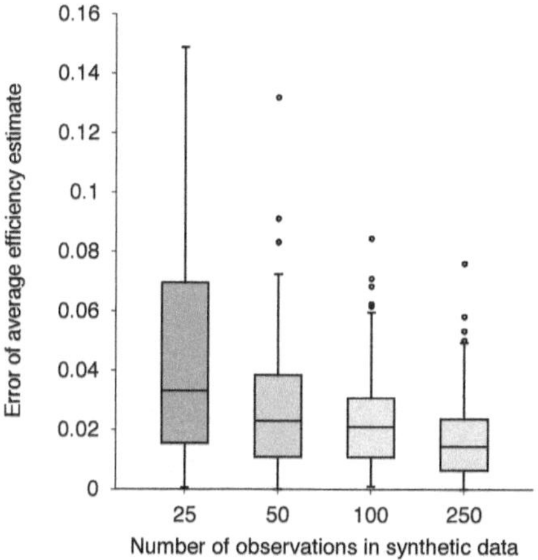

Figure 2.19 Estimation error of NMD efficiency. Each boxplot represents a distribution of average estimation errors in synthetic datasets. The x-axis represents the number of observations in each dataset. The y-axis represents the average estimation error across observations in each dataset. Bars in each box represents the median; top and bottom of each box represent the 25th and 75th percentiles; whiskers represent the 95% confidence interval, and points represent outliers. Each boxplot represents a distribution of average errors across 1000 synthetic datasets.

To generate NMD datasets, for each dataset, we generated randomized parameters α_e and β_e, characterizing the distribution of efficiencies for NMD. As we did previously, we generated individual distributions of AE for genes and sampled values of f from the distribution. We then randomly selected a value ϵ from the underlying distribution of NMD efficiency. We simulated the number of reads from each allele by drawing from a binomial distribution with the probability $p(f, e)$ (see Eqn. 5). Importantly, each observation in the dataset simulates the

51

variation of efficiency across genes, variants, and individuals, as well as statistical noise from the

small number of reads observed.

We evaluated our model's ability to infer NMD efficiency by calculating, for each

variant, the estimation error, defined as the absolute difference in efficiency between the

estimated ($\hat{\epsilon}$) and actual (ϵ) efficiencies (Figure 2.19). For even a modest number of observations

(N=25), we observed ~0.03 median error in the estimation of efficiency, decreasing to <0.02 for

datasets with more observations (N=100). Given the average efficiency of simulated NMD in

each dataset, these errors represent relative estimation errors less than ~5%.

BrainSpan expression data

We obtained the human brain RNA-Seq expression data from the BrainSpan Atlas of the

Developing Human Brain (brainspan.org) [84]. We used the BrainSpan project's developmental

transcriptome RNA-seq dataset, which includes tables summarizing the average expression level

in RPKM of human genes and their exons. RPKM values were quantile normalized across

samples.

Dosage-based model of phenotypic effect

Human genes likely differ in their contributions to specific phenotypes. Therefore, for

each gene with multiple LGD mutations in SSC, we estimated the IQ or VABS phenotype's

sensitivity to changes in gene dosage (i.e. phenotype dosage sensitivity or PDS). To that end, we

used least-squares linear regressions, regressing the observed phenotypic effects (y), defined as

the difference between the average neurotypical scores (100) and the proband's score, against the

relative expression of LGD targeted exons $\left(x_{\mathrm{rel}} = \frac{x_{\mathrm{exon}}}{x_{\mathrm{gene}}} \right)$. In each regression, we assumed that normal (wild type) gene dosage corresponds to a neurotypical score (100) and therefore fixed the

y-intercept at 0. The slope (s) of the fitted least-squares regression line provided an estimate of

the phenotypic sensitivity to gene dosage.

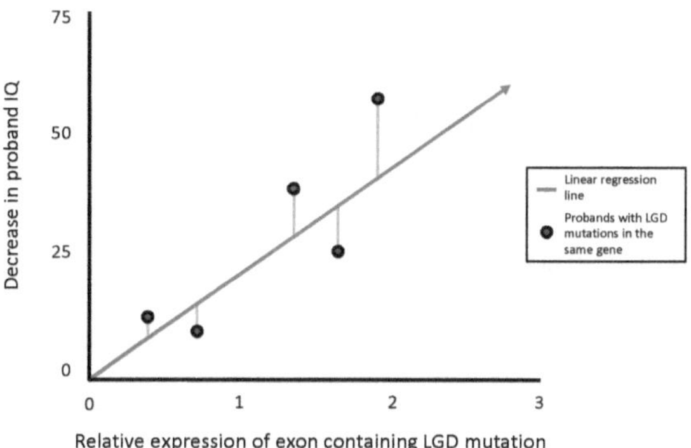

Figure 2.20 An illustration of the method we used to estimate phenotypic sensitivity to changes in the dosage of a gene. For each gene with multiple truncating mutations in SSC, we used least-squares linear regression to estimate the phenotypic sensitivity. We defined phenotypic sensitivity as the slope of the fitted regression between the relative expression of the target exon $\left(\frac{x_{exon}}{x_{gene}}\right)$ and the effect of the mutation, i.e. the corresponding proband's IQ compared to the average neurotypical value (100). Each blue point in the figure represents a proband with an LGD mutation in the same gene. The x-axis position indicates the relative expression the targeted exon. The y-axis position indicates the observed effect of the mutation on IQ. The red line shows the least-squares regression line.

To express these linear model parameters in terms of gene dosage, we used experimental

data from GTEx to model the average relationship between the relative expression of an exon

(x_{rel}) and the corresponding dosage changes observed due to LGD mutation(s) in that exon.

These predictions were made by averaging the dosage changes observed for GTEx LGD

mutations in exons with similar relative expression, defined as values within the δ half-width

interval $[x_{rel} - \delta, x_{rel} + \delta]$. We then averaged the observed dosage changes (Δx_{obs}) for GTEx

mutations in exons with relative expression values within the defined interval. Calculated in that way, predicted changes in dosage (Δx_{pred}) as a function of relative expression can be expressed

as:

$$\Delta x_{\text{pred}}(x_{\text{rel}}) = \frac{1}{|M|} \cdot \sum_{M} \Delta x_{\text{obs}} \qquad (10)$$

Where M is the set of LGD mutations in GTEx in exons with relative expression within ϵ of x_{rel}. The parameter δ was set to 0.05, which was chosen as the interval width for which estimated predicted dosage changes on average had SEM less than 1%.

We then analyzed phenotypic effects across multiple genes by normalizing $\left(y_{\text{norm}} = \frac{y}{s}\right)$ the effect of each LGD mutation by the PDS (s) of the affected gene, defined as the expected decrease in IQ (or VABS) due to a 10% change in gene dosage. To establish the statistical significance of the correlation between normalized phenotypic effects and changes in gene dosage, we used a permutation test. Specifically, we reassigned LGD mutations to randomly selected exons in the same gene, with the reassignment probability proportional to the length of each exon. Then, following the same normalization procedure, we computed the correlation between normalized phenotypic effects and relative exon expression in the randomly shuffled data. The distribution of the correlations observed in the permuted data was used to estimate empirical p-values.

Linear model-based predictions of the effects of LGD mutations

Based on the dosage sensitivity model described in the previous section, we performed leave-one-out predictions of the effect (y) of each LGD mutation on full-scale, nonverbal, and verbal IQ, defined as the difference between the observed IQ and the average neurotypical IQ (100). To predict the effect of each withheld mutation, we performed least-squares linear regression using all other mutation in the same gene. In each regression, the phenotypic impact of mutations was the dependent variable, and the relative expression $\left(x_{\text{rel}} = \frac{x_{\text{exon}}}{x_{\text{gene}}}\right)$ of target exons was the independent variable. We assumed that mutations with no effect on gene dosage would result in neurotypical IQs and fixed the y-intercept of each regression at 0. The fitted regression lines (with slope s) were used to predict the phenotypic impact of the withheld mutation $\left(y_{\text{pred}} = sx_{\text{rel}}\right)$. Prediction errors were calculated as the absolute difference between predicted and observed effects $\left(\left|y_{\text{pred}} - y\right|\right)$.

3 Autism phenotypes and the exon-intron structure of genes

3.1 Introduction

In the preceding investigations, we found a substantial correlation between the relative expression level of an exon harboring LGD variants and the changes in gene dosage due to nonsense-mediated decay (NMD) triggered by those variants. For truncating variants, the molecular effects at the transcript level (i.e. dosage loss due to NMD) are understood and, using the statistical methods we developed (see Section 2.3), can be quantified using RNA sequencing data. We hypothesized that across individuals, (1) consistent patterns of exon usage would lead to similar changes in gene dosage for LGD mutations in the same exon; and (2) similar dosage changes due to LGD mutations in the same exon would result in similar phenotypic consequences. To explore these hypotheses, we studied the phenotypes associated with LGD mutations in specific exons.

In the following results, we considered how the exon-intron structure of genes affects multiple important autism phenotypes, such as cognitive ability, adaptive behavior, fine motor skills, and coordination. We then investigated the molecular mechanisms potentially underlying our findings, including changes in gene dosage due to NMD and changes in the relative expression of splicing isoforms. Finally, we explored the relationships between the phenotypic consequences of LGD mutations and some functional properties of target exons, including position along gene and protein sequences, correspondence to sequences coding for protein domains, and inclusion in/exclusion from specific splicing isoforms.

3.2   Results

Exon-specific phenotypes for *de novo* LGD mutations in ASD

We first investigated the variability of cognitive phenotypes associated with *de novo*
LGD mutations in the same gene. Consistent with our preliminary analysis (Figure 0.3), we
found that the average IQ differences between probands with LGD mutations in the same gene
were only slightly smaller than the IQ differences between all pairs of probands (Figure 3.1).
Specifically, the mean pairwise differences for probands with mutations in the same gene were:
28.3 for FSIQ (~11% smaller compared to all pairs of ASD probands, Mann-Whitney U one-tail
test $p = 0.2$), 25.7 NVIQ (~12% smaller, $p = 0.14$), and 34.9 VIQ points (~1.1% smaller, $p =$
0.5).

We next considered the effect of exon-intron structure on IQ phenotypes. Specifically, we
investigated phenotypes resulting from truncating mutations affecting the same exon in unrelated
ASD probands; in this analysis, we took into account LGD mutations in the exon's coding
sequence as well as disruptions of the exon's flanking canonical splice sites, since such splice
site mutations should affect the same transcript isoforms (see Methods Figure 3.26).
Interestingly, the analysis of 16 unrelated ASD probands (8 pairs with LGD mutations in the
same exons) showed that they have strikingly more similar phenotypes (Figure 3.1, red bars)
compared to probands with LGD mutations in the same gene (Figure 3.1, dark green bars); same
exon FSIQ/NVIQ/VIQ average IQ difference 8.9, 8.3, 17.3 points, same gene average difference
28.3, 25.7, 34.9 points (Mann-Whitney U one-tail test $p = 0.003, 0.005, 0.016$). Because of well-
known gender differences in autism susceptibility [5, 85, 86], we also compared IQ differences
between probands of the same gender harboring truncating mutations in the same exon (Figure
3.1, orange bars) to IQ differences between probands of different genders; same gender

FSIQ/NVIQ/VIQ average difference 5.4, 7.2, 12.2; different gender average difference 14.7, 10, 25.7 (MWU one-tail test $P = 0.04, 0.29, 0.07$). Thus, stratification by gender further decreases the phenotypic differences between probands with LGD mutations in the same exon.

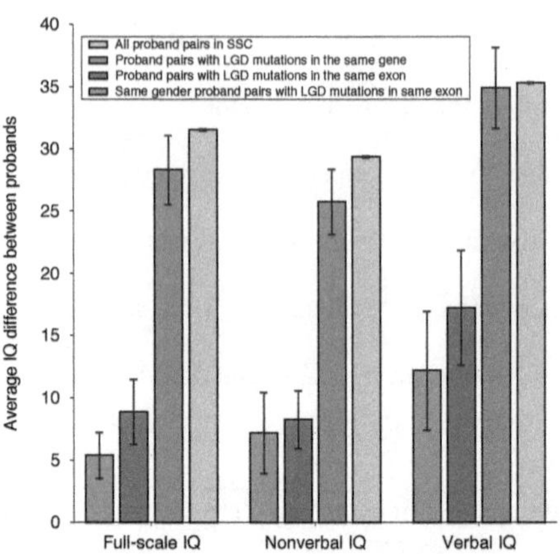

Figure 3.1 Average difference in IQs between SSC probands. From left to right, the sets of bars represent differences between full-scale, nonverbal, verbal IQs. Within each bar set, from right to left, the bars represent the average IQ difference between pairs of probands in the entire SSC cohort (light green), between probands with de novo LGD mutations in the same gene (dark green), between probands with de novo LGD mutations in the same exon (red), and between probands of the same gender and with de novo LGD mutations in the same exon (orange). Error bars represent the SEM.

We extended our analysis to adaptive behavior, measured using the Vineland Adaptive Behavior Scales (VABS) [87]. SSC probands with truncating mutations in the same exon exhibited more similar adaptive behavior abilities compared to probands with mutations in the same gene (Figure 3.2, left set of bars); VABS composite standard score difference of 4.7 versus 12.1 points (Mann-Whitney U one-tail test $p = 0.017$). In contrast, VABS differences between probands with truncating mutations in the same gene were not significantly different than for randomly paired probands (Figure 3.2); 12.1 versus 13.7 points (MWU one-tail test $p = 0.23$).

We also found similar patterns across specific categories of behavior (i.e. communication,

socialization, and daily living skills) quantified by VABS subscores (Figure 3.3).

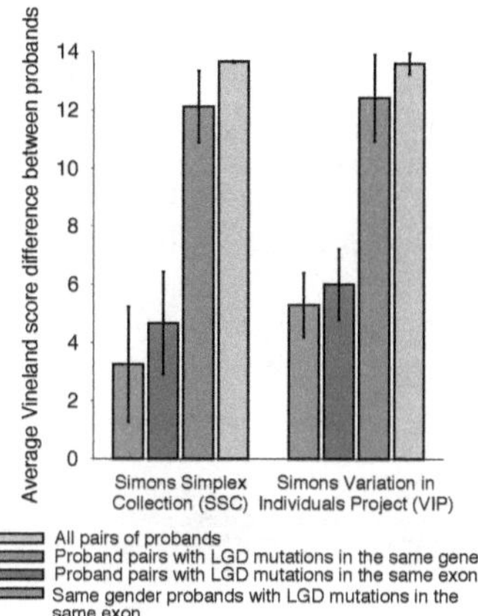

Figure 3.2 Vineland Adaptive Behavior Scales (VABS) score differences between probands using data from the Simons Simplex Collection (SSC) and the Simons Variation in Individuals Project (VIP). (a) Each bar shows the average difference in Vineland composite standard scores between pairs of probands in different groups. From right to left, bars represent differences between all pairs of probands in each cohort (light green), between probands with LGD mutations in the same gene (dark green), between probands with LGD mutations in the same exon (red), and between probands of the same gender with LGD mutations in the same exon (orange). Error bars represent the SEM.

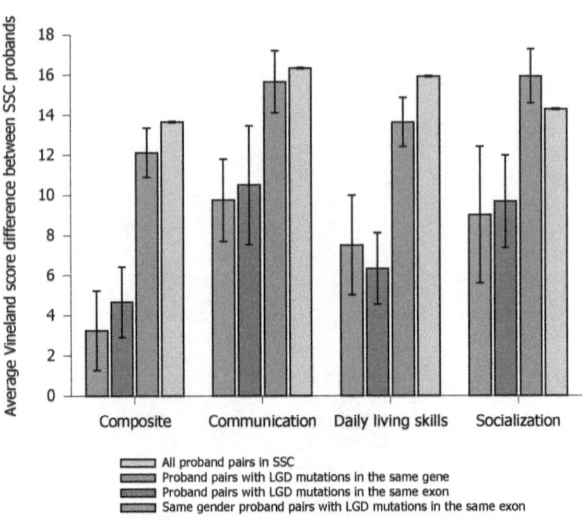

Figure 3.3 Average differences in adaptive behavior scores, i.e. Vineland Adaptive Behavior Scales, 2nd ed. (VABS), between probands in SSC. Each bar shows the average difference in VABS scores between pairs of probands. From left to right, bar groups represent differences in the composite score, and in communication, daily living skills (DLS), and socialization sub-scores. Within each bar group, bars represent, from right to left, the average score difference between all pairs of probands in the SSC cohort (light green), between probands with *de novo* LGD mutations in the same gene (dark green), between probands with *de novo* LGD mutations in the same exon (red), and between probands of the same gender and with *de novo* LGD mutations in the same exon (orange). Error bars represent the SEM.

To validate the observed phenotypic patterns, we analyzed an independently collected cohort of ASD probands from the ongoing Simons Variation in Individuals Project (VIP) [29]. The analyzed VIP dataset contained genetic information and VABS phenotypic scores for 41 individuals with *de novo* LGD mutations in 12 genes. Reassuringly, and consistent with our findings in SSC, probands from the VIP cohort with truncating *de novo* mutations in the same exon also exhibited strikingly more similar VABS phenotypic scores compared to probands with mutations in the same gene (Figure 3.2, right set of bars; Figure 3.4); VABS composite standard score difference 6.0 versus 12.4 (Mann-Whitney U one-tail test $p = 0.014$).

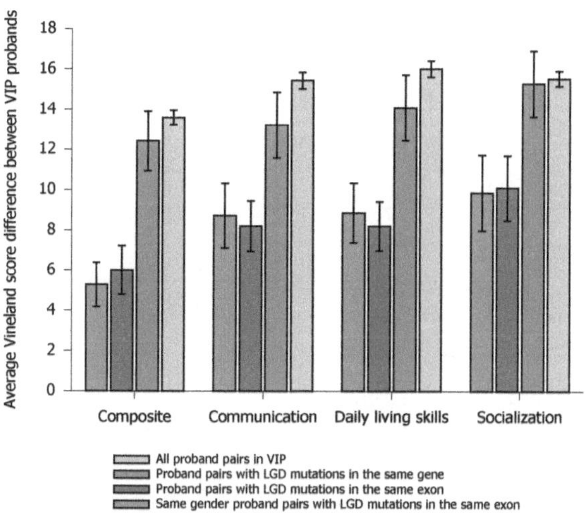

Figure 3.4 Average difference in Vineland adaptive behavior scores between probands in the Simons Variation in Individuals Project (VIP). Each bar shows the average difference in Vineland scores between pairs of probands. From left to right, bar groups represent differences in the composite standard score, and in communication, daily living skills (DLS), and socialization subscores. From right to left within each bar group, bars represent the average difference between all pairs of probands in the VIP cohort (light green), between probands with *de novo* LGD mutations in the same gene (dark green), between probands with *de novo* LGD mutations in the same exon (red), and between probands of the same gender with *de novo* LGD mutations in the same exon (orange). Error bars represent the SEM.

Importantly, the previous analyses describe the variability of individuals' phenotypes across multiple genes. To understand how these effects on phenotypes apply to specific genes, for each gene with multiple LGD mutations, we compared the phenotypic differences due to LGDs in the same exon and due to LGDs in different exons of the same gene. To obtain more statistical power for this analysis, we combined data from SSC and VIP and analyzed VABS scores, which were measured in both cohorts. The results demonstrated that phenotypic differences for mutations in the same exon were smaller, on average, for 7 out of 8 genes (Table 3.1). Furthermore, in agreement with other results presented in the paper, a paired statistical test across genes demonstrated that ASD phenotypes due to LGDs in the same exons were significantly more similar compared to LGDs in different exons of the same gene (Wilcoxon signed-rank one-tail $p = 0.012$).

Gene	LGDs in the same exon		LGDs in different exons of the same gene	
	Mean	N	Mean	N
ASXL3	6	3	11.2	15
CHD2	2	1	18	2
CHD8	11	1	12.8	20
DSCAM	1	1	12.5	2
DYRK1A	0	1	19.8	5
FOXP1	8.7	3	6.3	3
HIVEP2	6.7	3	13.7	3
SCN2A	6.5	2	13.8	14
P-value	P = 0.012, N = 8			

Table 3.1 Vineland (VABS) composite standard score differences between probands with LGD mutations in the same or different exons, stratified by gene. For each gene with multiple LGD mutations in multiple exons, we calculated the average difference in VABS scores between probands with LGDs in the same (left) and different exons (right) of the same gene. To compare effects across genes, we used a Wilcoxon signed-rank one-tail test to test whether scores for probands with mutations in the same exon were more similar than scores for probands with mutations in different exons of the same gene (Wilcoxon signed-rank one-tail $p = 0.012$).

Although we primarily focused on cognitive (IQ) and behavioral (VABS) phenotypes, we also analyzed several other important ASD phenotypes. We reasoned that the hypothesized underlying mechanisms – i.e. similar dosage changes from LGD mutations in the same exon – should lead to analogous results for other quantitative ASD phenotypes [24, 46]. Indeed, for LGD mutations predicted to lead to NMD, we observed similar patterns for several other key autism phenotypes. Probands with truncating mutations in the same exon displayed more similar fine motor skills; in the Purdue Pegboard Test, 1.2 versus 3.0 for the average difference in normalized tasks completed with both hands (MWU one-tail test $P = 0.02$; Figure 3.5; see Methods). Coordination scores in the Social Responsiveness Scale questionnaire were also more similar in probands with LGD mutations in the same exon compared to probands with mutations in the same gene; 0.6 versus 1.1 for the average difference in normalized response (MWU one-tail test $P = 0.05$; Figure 3.6).

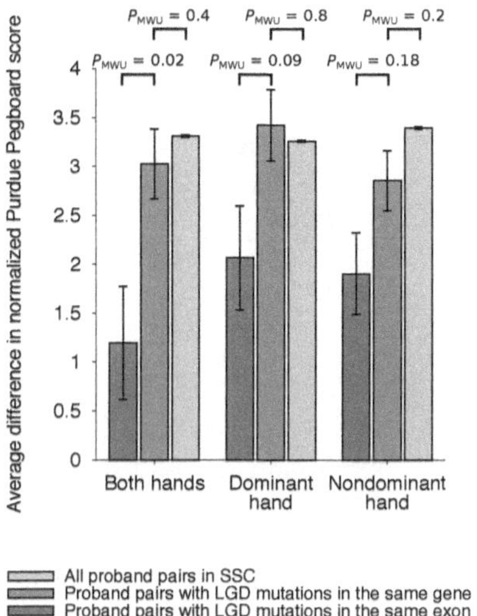

Figure 3.5 Average difference in Purdue Pegboard Test scores between pairs of ASD probands. From left to right, bar groups represent Purdue Pegboard Test scores for both hands, for the dominant hand, and for the non-dominant hand. Within each bar group, bars represent, from right to left, the average difference between all pairs of probands in SSC (light green), between pairs of probands with de novo LGD mutations in the same gene (dark green), and between pairs of probands with LGD mutations in the same exon (red). Purdue Pegboard scores were adjusted to account for probands' age and gender (see Methods). The statistical significances were calculated using Mann-Whitney U tests (PMWU). Error bars represent the SEM.

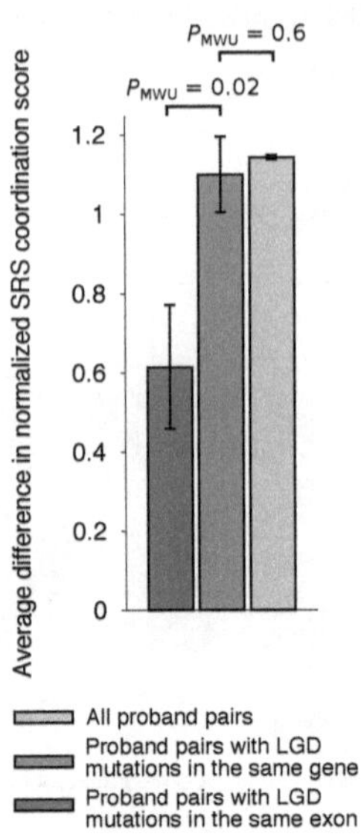

Figure 3.6 Average difference in Social Responsiveness Scales (SRS) coordination score between ASD probands. The bars represent, from right to left, all pairs of probands in SSC (light green), pairs of probands with de novo LGD mutations in the same gene (dark green), and between pairs of probands with LGD mutations in the same exon (red). SRS scores were adjusted to account for probands' age and gender (see Methods). The statistical significance was determined using Mann-Whitney U tests (PMWU). Error bars represent the SEM.

We then investigated the relationship between background genetic variation in individuals and the phenotypic effects of *de novo* LGD mutations in specific exons. Accordingly, we separately analyzed probands from trio families (i.e. families without unaffected siblings). In these probands, the enrichment of LGD mutations is likely to be substantially lower, and the contribution from genetic background larger [88]. Interestingly, when affected by LGD mutations in the same exon, probands from sequenced trio families varied significantly (~2 times) more in IQ phenotypes than probands from quad families (Figure 3.7), suggesting that probands' genetic backgrounds additionally affect the phenotypic consequences of mutations.

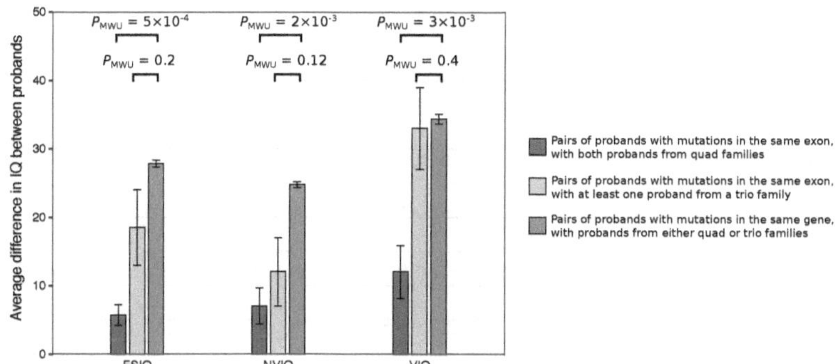

Figure 3.7 Average IQ differences between SSC probands from quad and trio ASD families. Quad families have a single affected child among with one or multiple unaffected; trio families have an affected child with no siblings. From left to right, differences are shown for full-scale IQ (FSIQ), nonverbal IQ (NVIQ), and verbal IQ (VIQ) scores. For each score, bars represent the average IQ difference between probands with *de novo* LGD mutations in the same gene (dark green), between pairs of probands with mutations in the same exon and with at least one proband from a trio family (light green), and between probands from quad families with mutations in the same exon (purple). The statistical significance was calculated using Mann-Whitney U test (P_{MWU}). Error bars indicate the SEM.

As a negative control, we analyzed probands with synonymous mutations in the same

exon. Reassuringly, such probands were as phenotypically diverse as random pairs of probands

(FSIQ, NVIQ, VIQ Mann-Whitney U on-tail test $p = 0.93, 0.97, 0.95$; Figure 3.8). Interestingly,

when we analyzed missense mutations in the same exon, we also did not see a significant

decrease in variability between affected probands (MWU one-tail test $p = 0.8, 0.5, 0.8$; Figure

3.9), potentially because their effects on protein stability and function may significantly vary

within the coding sequence of a single exon. These results suggest that the underlying

mechanisms that explain our observations are specific to LGD mutations.

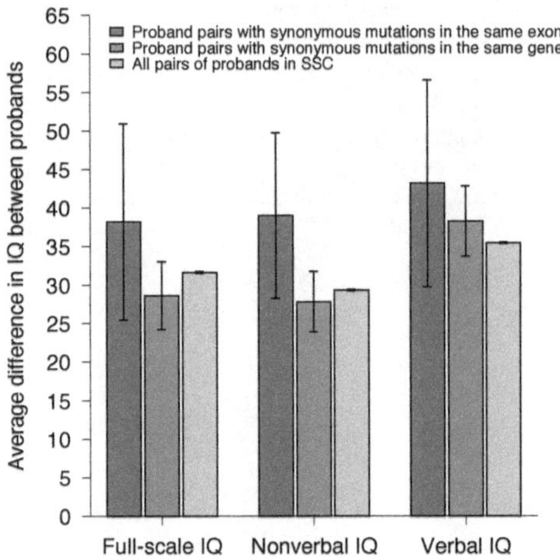

Figure 3.8 The average differences in IQ between probands with synonymous mutations in the same gene or the same exon. Each bar represents the average IQ difference between all pairs of probands in the SSC cohort (light green), between pairs of probands with synonymous mutations in the same gene (dark green), and between pairs of probands with synonymous mutations in the same exon (red). From left to right, sets of bars represent differences for full-scale, nonverbal, and verbal IQs. Error bars represent the SEM.

66

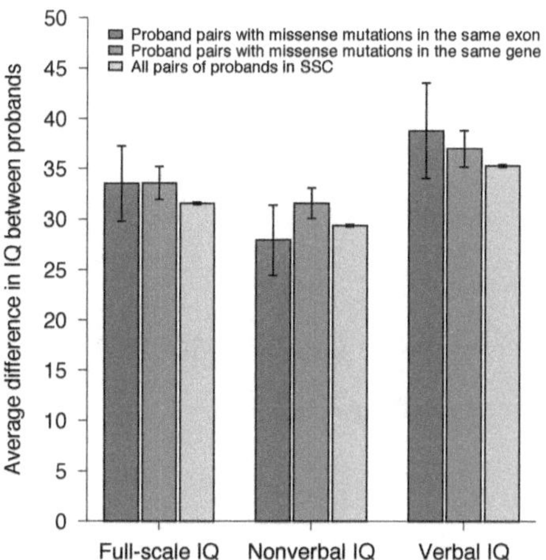

Figure 3.9 Average difference in IQ between probands with missense mutations in the same gene or the same exon. Each bar represents the average IQ difference between all pairs of probands in the SSC cohort (light green), between pairs of probands with missense mutations in the same gene (dark green), and between missense mutations in the same exon (red). Error bars represent the SEM.

To explain the similarity of phenotypes resulting from LGD mutations in the same exon, we hypothesized that truncating mutations in the same exon usually affect, due to nonsense-mediated decay (NMD) [64], the expression of exactly the same sets of splicing isoforms. Therefore, such mutations should lead to similar phenotypes, both through similar decreases in overall gene dosage and similar perturbations to the relative expression of the same transcriptional isoforms. To evaluate this mechanistic model, we used data from the Genotype and Tissue Expression (GTEx) Consortium [76, 77], which collected exome sequencing and corresponding human tissue-specific gene expression data from hundreds of individuals and across multiple tissues. Using ~4,400 LGD variants in coding regions and corresponding RNA-seq data, we compared the expression changes resulting from LGD variants in the same and different exons of the same gene (Figure 3.10). Specifically, for each truncating variant, we analyzed allele-specific read counts [65] and then developed and used a novel empirical Bayes approach to estimate the effects of NMD on gene expression (see Chapter 2).

This analysis confirmed that the average gene dosage changes for individuals with LGD variants in the same exon were ~7 times more similar compared to individuals with LGD variants in different exons of the same gene (Figure 3.10a); 2.2% versus 17.3% average difference in the decrease of overall gene dosage (Mann-Whitney U one-tail test $p < 2\times10^{-16}$). Moreover, by analyzing GTEx data for each human tissue separately, we found that, across all tissues, LGD variants in the same exons led to drastically more similar dosage changes of target genes (Figure 3.10a).

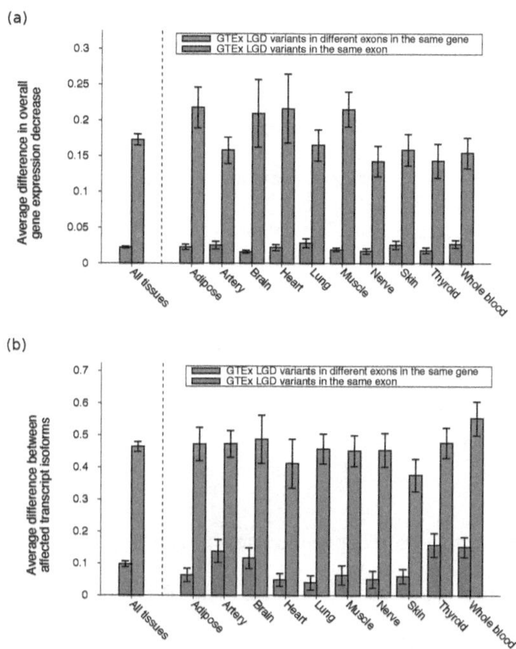

Figure 3.10 Gene expression changes across human tissues due to LGD variants in the same exon and in the same gene but different exons. Expression changes (decreases) due to LGD variants were calculated based on data from the Genotype and Tissue Expression (GTEx) Consortium. (a) Bars represent the average difference across the GTEx cohort in overall gene expression changes induced by distinct LGD variants in the same exon (red) and in the same gene but different exons (blue). Error bars represent the SEM. (b) Bars represent the average difference across the GTEx cohort in isoform-specific expression changes induced by distinct LGD variants in the same exon (red) and in the same gene but different exons (blue). Differences in expression changes across transcriptional isoforms were quantified using the angular distance metric between vectors representing isoform-specific expression changes (see Methods). Error bars represent the SEM.

Distinct splicing isoforms have different functional properties [89, 90], and based on our previous analyses, we hypothesized LGD variants may affect phenotypes not only through NMD-induced changes in overall gene dosage, considered above, but also by altering the relative expression levels of all isoforms in a similar way. To analyze changes in the relative expression of isoforms, we next used GTEx variants to quantify the effects of NMD on each isoform of a gene. To compare isoform-specific expression changes in the same gene, we calculated an angular distance metric between vectors representing dosage changes for each isoform (see Methods). This analysis demonstrated that changes in relative isoform expression are also significantly (~5 fold) more similar for LGD variants in the same exon compared to variants in different exons of the same gene (Figure 3.10b); 0.1 versus 0.46 for the average angular distance between isoform-specific expression vectors (Mann-Whitney U one-tail test $p < 2 \times 10^{-16}$). These results were also consistent across tissues (Figure 3.10b). Overall, the analyses of GTEx data demonstrate that both overall changes in gene dosage and changes in the relative expression levels of different isoforms are substantially more similar for truncating mutations in same exons.

We sought to further confirm our results using *in vitro* experimental measurements. To that end, we used data from a previously published CRISPR/Cas9-based genetic editing experiment in HAP1 cell lines [67, 68]. In the experiment, nearly all possible single nucleotide variants (~3,900 SNVs) were introduced across entire sequences of target exons in the BRCA1 gene. The effect of each LGD mutation on gene dosage was calculated by estimating the mRNA expression level for each cell affected by the LGD mutation. In our analysis, we found that gene dosage varied approximately twice as much for LGD mutations in different exons versus LGD mutations in the same exon; 0.17 versus 0.32 mean difference in dosage due to mutations in the same exon and different exons, respectively; Mann-Whitney U one-tail test $p < 2.2 \times 10^{-16}$ (Figure 3.11). These results experimentally validated our analyses of GTEx expression data and were consistent with the analysis phenotypic data in SSC and VIP.

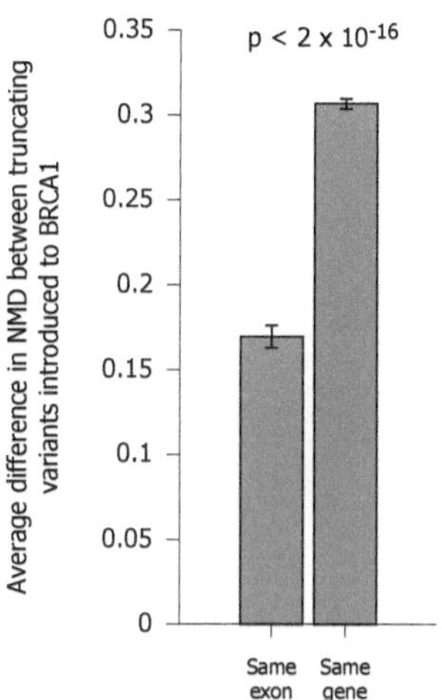

Figure 3.11 Differences in the effects of NMD between LGD mutations in the same exon and LGDs in the same gene (BRCA1), but not necessarily the same exon. Bars represent pairs of LGD mutations in the same exon and pairs of LGD mutations in the same gene. The y-axis represents the average difference in dosage change between LGD mutations in the same exon or the same gene. Change in dosage due to NMD were calculated by comparing the expression level of BRCA1 for cells with LGD mutations to the average expression level for cells with synonymous mutations. Annotations represent the Mann-Whitney one-tail test p-value. Error bars represent the SEM.

Given the strong selective pressure against LGD mutations in exons with higher relative expression, we then asked, at the population level, if exons expressed at similar levels would have similar intolerance to LGD mutations. To investigate, we used ultra-rare (UR) variants, defined as variants observed only once in a sequenced population, in the Exome Aggregation Consortium (ExAC) dataset to estimate the intolerance of exons to LGD mutations. Specifically, we calculated for each exon the ratio of UR LGD variants to UR synonymous variants. When we compared differences in the percent usage of exons and the intolerance of exons to LGD variants, we indeed found that different exons with similar usage indeed had similar intolerance to LGD mutations (Mann-Kendall one tail test $p < 2{\times}10^{-16}$; Figure 3.12). For example, exons that differed less than 10% in three times less variability (0.05 vs. 0.15) in intolerance compared to exons with differences in usage >50%.

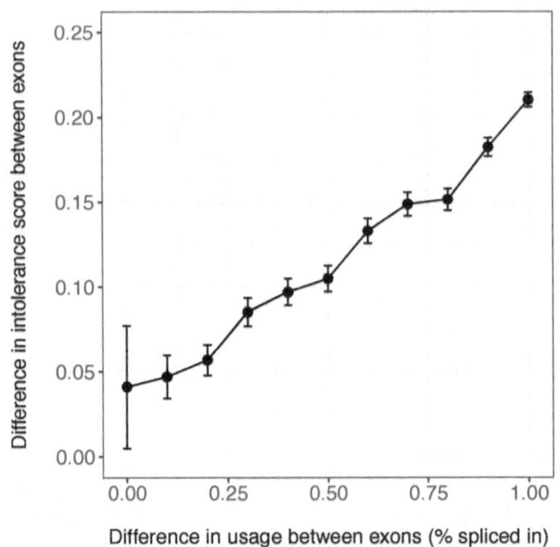

Figure 3.12 Similarity in intolerance to LGD mutations for exons with similar dosage. For each pair of exons in a gene, we compared their differences in usage (calculated as the absolute difference in percent spliced-in or PSI) and their intolerance to LGD mutations. The x-axis represents the difference in PSI between exons; from left to right, points represent comparisons between exons with increasing differences in usage. The y-axis represents the average difference in intolerance score between exons. Intolerance scores were defined as the ratio of ultra-rare (UR), i.e. observed only once in a sequencing population, LGD variants to UR synonymous variants in the exon. Error bars represent the SEM.

We then used exons' intolerance to LGD variation to estimate the relative contributions to evolutionary selection of overall gene-level dosage changes versus changes in the relative expression of isoform. When we compared intolerance scores between exons affecting exactly the same isoforms versus exons with similar dosage but affecting different isoforms, we found that the similarity in usage explained 45% of the variability in selection across exons, while the targeting of specific isoforms contributed ~55% of the variability (Figure 3.13).

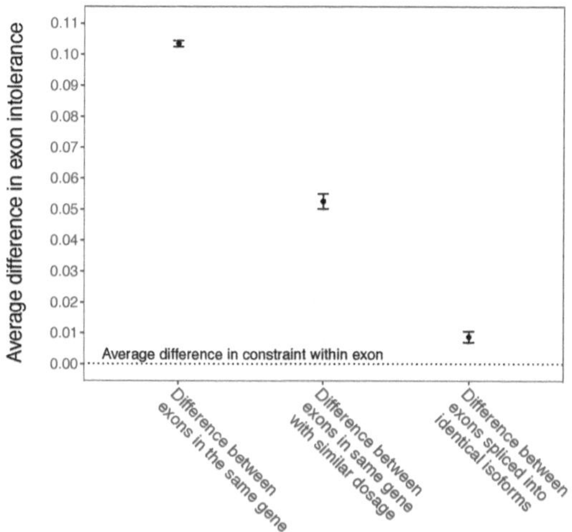

Figure 3.13 Relative contributions of gene- and isoform-level dosage changes to exon intolerance. From left to right, points represent the difference in intolerance score between exons in the same gene, between exons in the same gene with similar percent spliced-in (difference in PSI ≤ 0.1), and between exons spliced into exactly the same transcriptional isoforms. Intolerance scores were defined as the ratio of ultra-rare, i.e. observed only once, LGD variants to UR synonymous variants in the ExAC dataset. Values were normalized to the average difference in scores within an exon. Error bars represent the SEM.

Phenotypic consequences of LGD mutations across gene and protein sequences

Given the similarity of phenotypes resulting from LGD mutations in the same exon, we investigated whether LGD mutations in neighboring exons would also produce similar phenotypes. Notably, the patterns of phenotypic similarity between probands only extended to mutations in the same exon. The average IQ differences between SSC probands with LGD mutations in neighboring exons were not significantly different compared to mutations in non-neighboring exons (MWU one-tail test $p = 0.6, 0.18, 0.8$; Figure 3.14). Similarly, in the independent VIP cohort, LGD mutations in neighboring exons also did not result in more similar

73

behavior phenotypes (VABS composite standard score average difference 13.6 points; MWU one-tail test $p = 0.6$) than LGD mutations in the same gene.

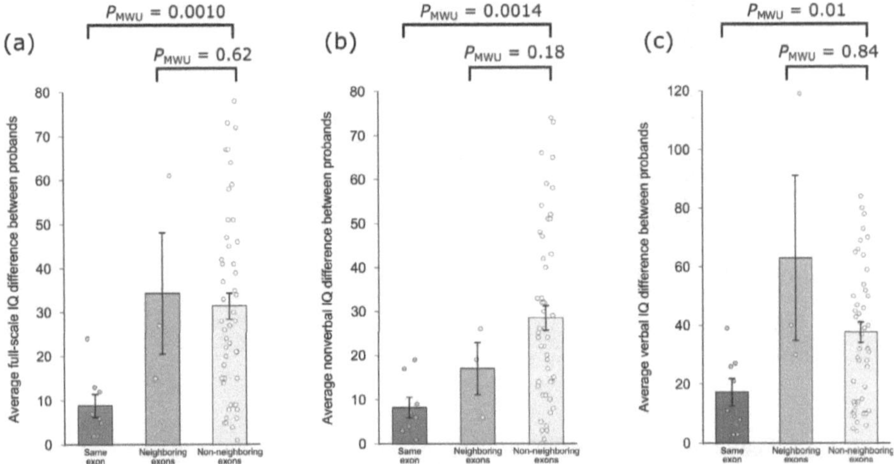

Figure 3.14 The average IQ differences between probands with LGD mutations in the same exon, in neighboring exons of the same gene, and in non-neighboring exons of the same gene. Plots represent (a) full-scale IQ (FSIQ), (b) nonverbal IQ (NVIQ), and (c) verbal IQ (VIQ) scores. Each overlaid point represents a pair of probands with LGD mutations in the same exon, in neighboring exons, or in non-neighboring exons. The y-axis represents the IQ difference between affected probands. The statistical significance was determined using Mann-Whitney U tests (PMWU). Error bars represent the SEM.

To understand more generally how the proximity of LGD mutations affects proband phenotypes, we asked whether LGD mutations at similar locations in gene sequence were associated with more similar proband phenotype (Figure 3.15). Consistent with our exon-level findings, IQ differences between probands with LGD mutations closer than 1000 base pairs apart were indeed significantly smaller than the IQ differences between probands with more distant mutations; ≤1 kbp FSIQ/NVIQ/VIQ average difference 11.5, 10.4, 20.6 points; >1 kbp average difference 31.4, 28.6, 37.5 points (MWU one-tail test $p = 0.002, 0.005, 0.01$). However, across the entire range of nucleotide distances between LGD mutations in the same genes, we did not observe either a significant correlation or a monotonic relationship between IQ differences and mutation proximity (FSIQ/NVIQ/VIQ Spearman's ρ = 0.09, 0.1, 0.03, p = 0.5, 0.4, 0.8; one-tail

Mann-Kendall test p = 0.5, 0.3, 0.6).

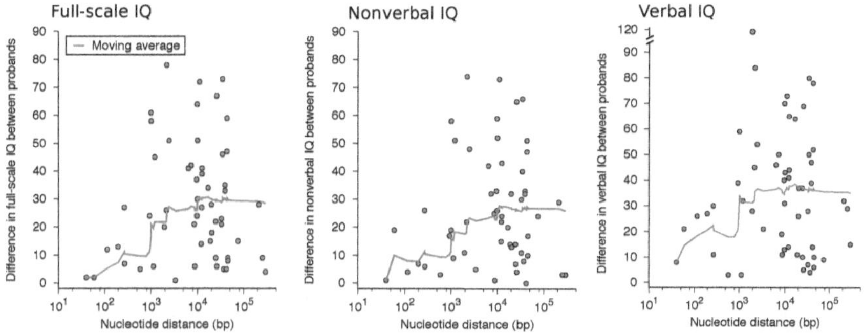

Figure 3.15 IQ differences between pairs of probands with de novo LGD mutations in the same gene. Each point in the figures corresponds to a pair of probands from the SSC cohort with de novo LGD mutations in the same gene. The x-axis represents the nucleotide distance between LGD mutations. The y-axis represents the absolute difference in IQs (full-scale, nonverbal, or verbal IQ) between affected probands. Moving averages are shown in red.

We next explored the relationship between phenotypic similarity and the proximity of

truncating mutations in the corresponding protein sequences. This analysis revealed that

probands with LGD mutations in the same exon often had similar IQs, despite being affected by

truncating mutations separated by scores to hundreds of amino acids in protein sequence (Figure

3.16). Furthermore, we found probands with LGD mutations in the same exon to be more

phenotypically similar than probands with LGD mutations separated by comparable amino acid

distances in the same protein sequence but not necessarily in the same exon (FSIQ/NVIQ/VIQ

distance-matched permutation test p = 0.010, 0.002, 0.018; Figure 3.17; see Methods).

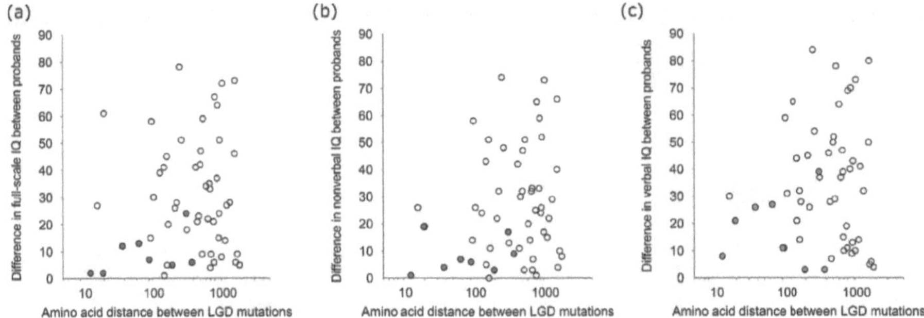

Figure 3.16 Amino acid distance between LGD mutations in protein sequence versus the IQ differences between corresponding probands. From left to right, plots show differences in (a) full-scale IQ (FSIQ), (b) nonverbal IQ (NVIQ), and (c) verbal IQ (VIQ) scores. Each point in the figures corresponds to a pair of probands affected by de novo LGD mutations in the same gene. The x-axis represents the amino acid distance between LGD mutations, and the y-axis represents the absolute difference between the probands' IQs. Open (white) points correspond to pairs of probands with LGD mutations in different exons of the same genes; filled (colored) points correspond to pairs of probands with mutations in the same exon of the same genes.

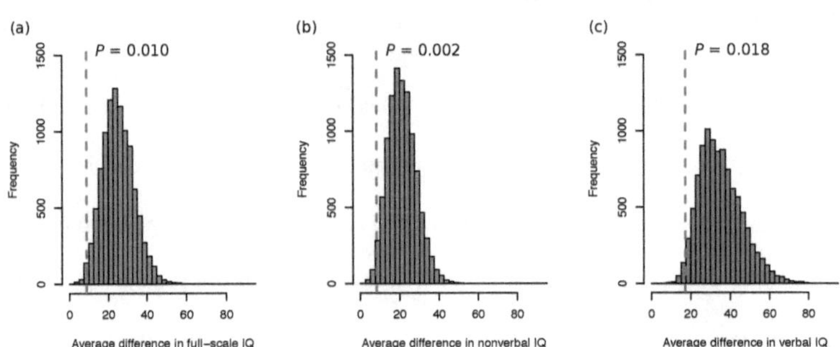

Figure 3.17 Simulated null distributions of the average IQ difference between probands with de novo LGD mutations in the same gene and with similar distances in the corresponding protein sequence. From left to right, histograms show the distribution of average differences for (a) full-scale IQ (FSIQ), (b) nonverbal IQ (NVIQ), and (c) verbal IQ (VIQ) scores across the sampled null distribution trials (N=10,000). The histograms show the null trial frequencies of the average IQ differences (x-axes) between pairs of probands with mutations in the same gene, where mutations were separated by amino acid distances similar to the ones empirically observed between LGD mutations in the same exon (see Methods). The red dashed lines represent the observed average IQ differences between probands with LGD mutations in the same exon.

Using data from both SSC and VIP, we similarly investigated whether the similarity of VABS scores was due to the presence of mutations in the same exon, rather than proximity of truncating mutations within the corresponding protein sequence. Indeed, LGD mutations in the same exon often resulted in similar adaptive behavior abilities even when the corresponding mutations were separated by hundreds of amino acids (Figure 3.18). By comparing mutations in the same exon to mutations separated by similar amino acid distances in the same protein but not necessarily the same exon, we confirmed that probands with mutations in the same exon were significantly more phenotypically similar (permutation test $p = 3 \times 10^{-4}$; Figure 3.19; see Methods).

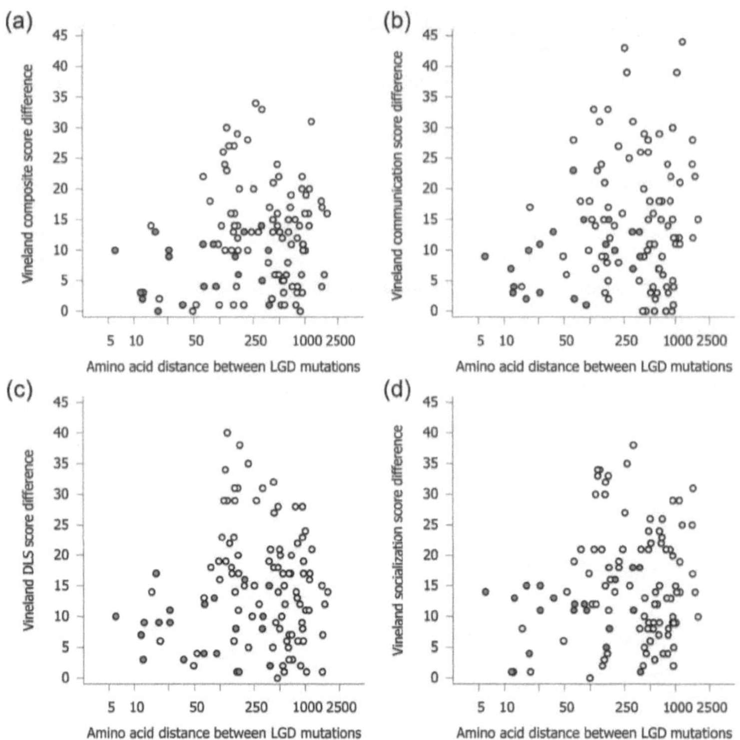

Figure 3.18 Amino acid distance between LGD mutations in the same protein versus the differences in Vineland (VABS) score between probands; data from the SSC and VIP cohorts were combined. Clockwise from top left, plots show differences in VABS (a) composite standard score, and (b) communication, (c) daily living skills (DLS), and (d) socialization subscores. In the figures, each point corresponds to a pair of probands affected by *de novo* LGD mutations in the same gene. The *x*-axis represents the amino acid distance between LGD mutations, and the *y*-axis represents the difference between the affected probands' VABS scores. Open (white) points correspond to proband pairs with mutations in different exons of the same gene; filled (colored) points correspond to pairs with mutations in the same exon.

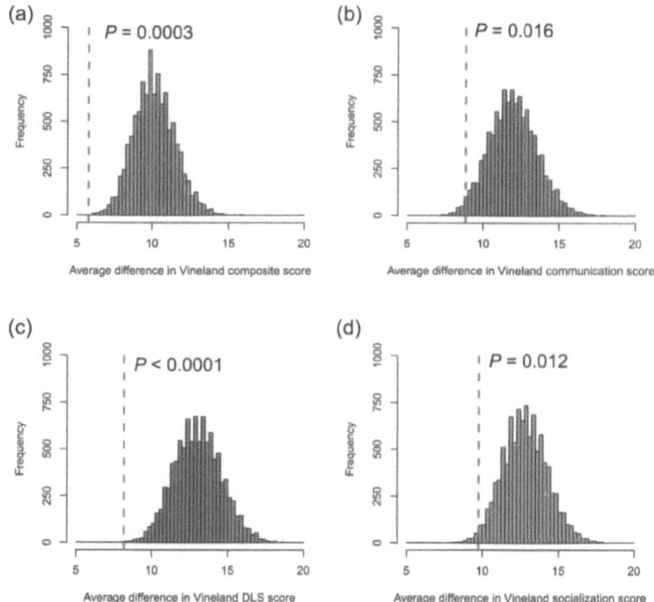

Figure 3.19 Simulated null distributions of the average Vineland (VABS) score difference between ASD probands (from the combined SSC and VIP cohort) with *de novo* LGD mutations in the same gene and separated by similar distances in corresponding protein sequence. Clockwise from top left, histograms represent the distribution of average differences in VABS score for (a) the composite standard score, and for the (b) communication, (c) daily living skills (DLS), and (d) socialization subscores. Each value in the histogram represents the average Vineland score difference between pairs of probands with mutations in the same gene and with protein amino acid distances similar to the distances empirically observed for LGD mutations in the same exon (see Methods). The red dashed lines represent the observed average score differences between probands with mutations in the same exon.

We also investigated whether *de novo* mutations truncating a larger fraction of protein sequences resulted, on average, in more severe phenotypes. Surprisingly, this analysis showed no significant correlations between the fraction of truncated protein and the severity of intellectual phenotypes (FSIQ/NVIQ/VIQ Pearson's R = 0.05, 0.05, 0.06; p = 0.35, 0.35, 0.28; Figure 3.20). Across both SSC and VIP, the fraction of truncated proteins also did not show significant correlation with the VABS scores of affected probands (Pearson's R = -0.08, p = 0.7). We also did not find any significant biases in the distribution of truncating *de novo* mutations across

79

protein sequences compared with the distribution of synonymous *de novo* mutations

(Kolmogorov-Smirnov two-tail test $p = 0.9$; Figure 3.21). It is possible that the lack of the

correlation between phenotypic impact and the fraction of truncated sequence is due to the

averaging of effects across many proteins with diverse functions. Therefore, for genes with

recurrent mutations, we used a paired test to investigate whether truncating a larger fraction of

the same protein sequence led to more severe phenotypes. This analysis also showed no

substantial phenotypic difference due to LGD mutations truncating different fractions of the

same protein (average NVIQ difference 0.24 points; Wilcoxon signed-ranked one-tail test $p =$

0.44).

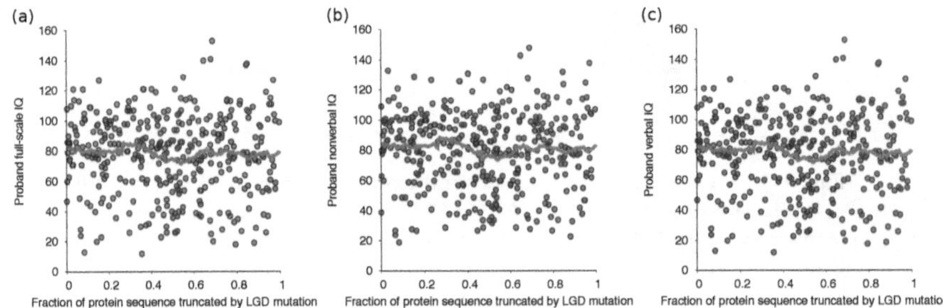

Figure 3.20 Relative fraction of protein sequence truncated by LGD mutations versus proband IQs. Each point corresponds to a single proband in SSC affected by an LGD mutation. From left to right, the plots show (a) full-scale IQ (FSIQ), (b) nonverbal IQ (NVIQ), and (c) verbal IQ (VIQ) scores. The x-axis represents the fraction of protein amino acid sequence (i.e. fraction from the first amino acid) truncated by the LGD mutation. The y-axis represents the corresponding proband's IQ score. Red lines represent moving averages of the data.

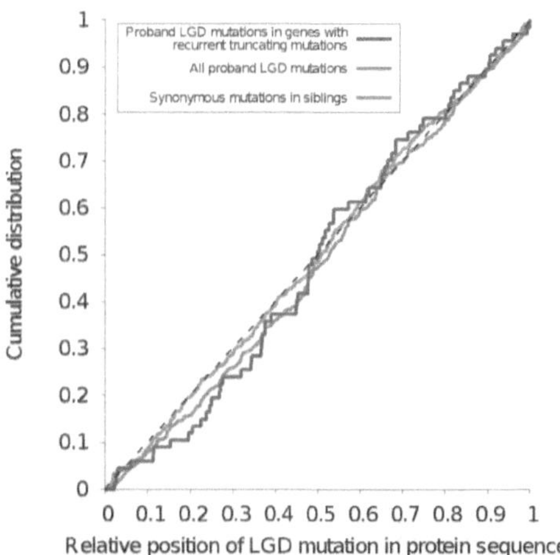

Figure 3.21 Cumulative distributions of the relative amino acid positions of de novo LGD mutations. Each line represents the cumulative distribution of the relative protein sequence positions (i.e. fraction of the total sequence length from the first amino acid) for LGD mutations in genes with multiple truncating mutations in SSC (red), for all LGD mutations in SSC (orange), and for synonymous mutations in unaffected siblings in SSC (blue).

Phenotypic consequences of LGDs affecting functional coding sequences

Mutations close to each other in protein sequence, such as mutations in the same exon, are likely to affect the same protein domains. To separate the effect of losing similar domains from the effect of targeting the same exon, we used the Pfam database [91] to identify mutations truncating the same protein domain (see Methods Figure 3.27). Mutations in different exons, even when truncating the same protein domain, resulted in very different phenotypes, i.e. phenotypes as different as due to two random LGD mutations in the same gene (Figure 3.22). We observed consistent results for both IQs (average NVIQ difference = 28.1; Figure 3.22a) and Vineland scores (average VABS composite score difference = 14.1; Figure 3.22b).

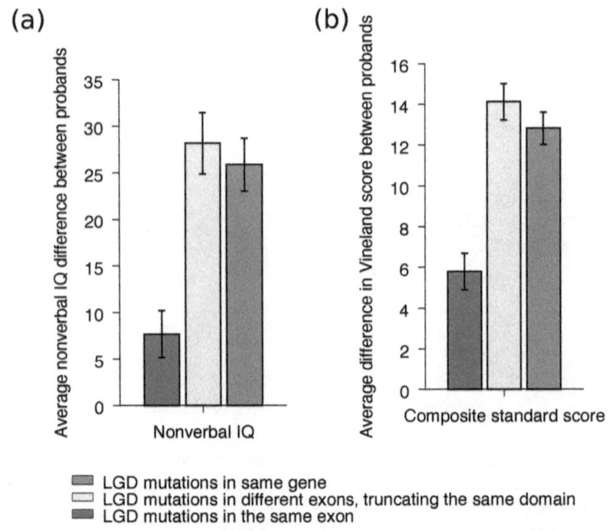

Figure 3.22 Average phenotypic differences between probands with LGD mutations truncating the same protein domain. Bars represent the average difference in (a) nonverbal IQ or (b) Vineland composite standard scores between pairs of probands with LGD mutations affecting: the same gene (dark green); different exons, but truncating the same domain (grey); or the same exon (red). Error bars represent the SEM.

We also investigated whether mutations that truncate more protein domains lead to more severe phenotypes. Interestingly, for both NVIQ and VABS composite scores, we found no significant correlation between phenotype severity and the number of protein domains lost due to truncating mutations (NVIQ Pearson's R = -0.054, Spearman's ρ = 0.016; VABS Pearson's R = -0.012, Spearman's ρ = 0.031; Figure 3.23).

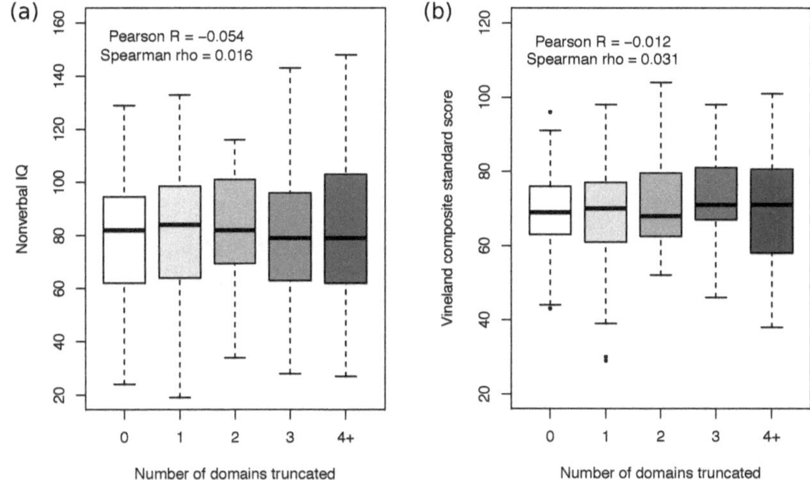

Figure 3.23 Relationship between number of domains lost due to LGD mutations and proband phenotypes. Boxplots represents the distribution of (a) nonverbal IQ or (b) Vineland (VABS) scores for probands affected by LGD mutations. Within each panel, from left to right, probands are grouped by increasing number of protein domains truncated by LGD mutations. Lines in the middle of each box represent median scores, the top and bottom of each box represents the 25th and 75th percentiles respectively, and the whiskers represent the 5th and 95th percentiles. Outliers, defined as values more than 1.5 IQRs from the median, are plotted as individual points.

Different splicing isoforms of a gene can have different functional properties [89, 90].

Moreover, even genes with dozens of isoforms express a dominant isoform that captures a large

fraction (>30%) of total gene expression [92]. Consequently, we investigated whether the

similarity of phenotypes resulting from LGD mutations in the same exon could be attributed to

truncation of a single, functionally important isoform. By using the APPRIS database to identify

major isoforms [93], we found that LGD mutations affecting a common major isoform led to

significantly higher (2-3 times) phenotypic diversity compared to mutations in the same exon

(Figure 3.24). The likely reason for this result is that truncating mutations in the same exon do not just affect a single isoform, but affect, in a similar way, the whole set of isoforms containing

the target exon.

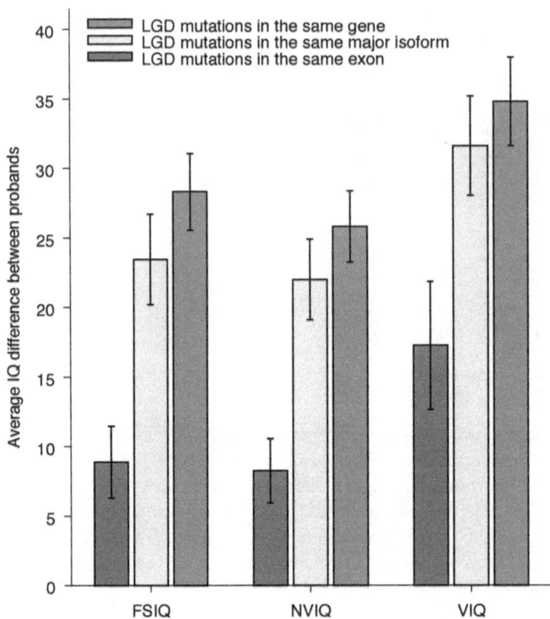

Figure 3.24 IQ differences between pairs of probands with mutations affecting the same principal isoform of a gene. Each bar represents the average difference in IQ between pairs of probands with LGD mutations: in the same gene (dark green), in the same major isoform (grey), or in the same exon (red). Major isoforms for each gene were identified using the APPRIS database. Error bars represent the standard error of the mean.

To understand the phenotypic consequences of mutations affecting multiple common

isoforms, we calculated the correlation between probands' phenotypic similarity and the fraction

of shared isoforms that are affected by the mutations. We note that our current knowledge of

major human gene isoforms is quite incomplete. Despite this, based on isoform annotations in

Ensembl [87], we indeed found a significant correlation between the fraction of shared isoforms

84

and similarity of NVIQ and VABS phenotypes; Spearman's R = -0.21, -0.19; p = 0.02, 0.006; for NVIQ and VABS, respectively.

We then investigated whether the phenotypic consequences of an LGD mutation in an exon could be explained by its evolutionary conservation. To that end, we correlated the evolutionary conservation of exons harboring LGD mutations with the IQ phenotypes of the affected probands. Using several different measures of evolutionary conservation, including GERP scores [94], PhyloP [95], and PhastCons [96], we found relatively weak correlations between the conservation of the exon and the probands' IQs (NVIQ versus GERP/PhyloP/PhastCons scores, Pearson's R = -0.13, -0.14, -0.03; Figure 3.25). Thus, differences in the evolutionary conservation of target exons can explain at most ~1-2% of the phenotypic variance across individuals.

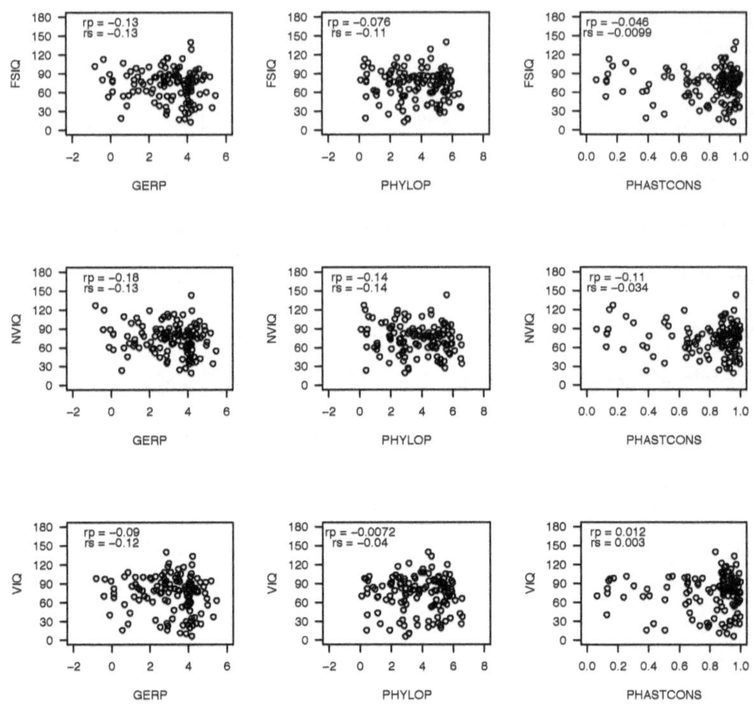

Figure 3.25 Evolutionary conservation of exons versus proband IQ phenotypes. Each point in the scatterplots represents an SSC proband affected by an LGD mutation. In each panel, the x-axes represent the evolutionary conservation of exons harboring LGD mutations. Evolutionary conservation was quantified (from left to right columns) using GERP, phyloP, or PhastCons scores. The y-axes represent (from top to bottom rows) the full-scale, nonverbal, or verbal IQ score for probands affected by the mutations. Pearson's R (rp) and Spearman's rho (rs) are given for each plot.

3.3   Methods

We used exome sequencing and phenotypic data available in the Simons Simplex

Collection (SSC) [28]. Specifically, *de novo* LGD mutations were obtained from Iossifov *et al.*

[8], and phenotypic data were obtained from Prepared Phenotype Dataset (v15) available through

the SFARI Base online data portal (sfari.org/resources/sfari-base). From the Simons Variation in

Individuals Project (VIP) [29], we analyzed *de novo* LGD mutations and and phenotypes the

Simons VIP Phase 2 Single Gene Dataset v4.0, also available on SFARI Base.

SSC and SVIP include ASD probands of both genders spanning a broad range of ages

and phenotypic abilities. While some phenotypes, such as IQ and VABS scores, are already

normalized based on gender and age, other phenotypes are provided as raw scores that vary with

the age and/or gender of the proband. To account for the effects of age and gender, we adjusted

raw scores for such unnormalized phenotypes. Following an approach previously used by Buja,

et al. [97], we adjusted phenotypic scores using linear regression. Specifically, using phenotypic

scores from all probands, we performed a multivariate linear regression for each raw score, with

age and gender as independent regression parameters. We used a binary variable (taking value 0

for male or 1 for female) to capture mean differences across genders. We then used the

regression residuals as adjusted scores for comparing proband phenotypes.

Notably, while the SSC and VIP datasets does not provide the exact age of probands at

the time when each specific phenotype was collected, we approximated the probands' ages by using the age at which the Autism Diagnostic Observation Schedule was administered (database

column "age at ADOS").

Registration of splice site mutations to exons

To study the effects of exon-intron structure, we considered LGD mutations, including

nonsense, frameshift, and splice site mutations, either in the same exon or in different exons of a

a target gene. Splice site mutations, which affect intronic sequences, were assigned to the

adjacent exon, rather than the target intron. Such splice site mutations should affect the same

transcript isoforms as coding sequence mutations in the flanked exon (Figure 3.26).

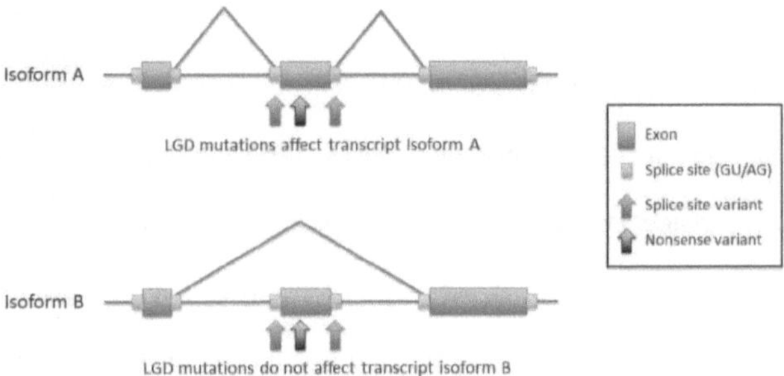

Figure 3.26 Illustration showing an example of LGD mutations affecting either of two
transcriptional isoforms of a gene. Exons are represented by blue rectangles, their flanking canonical
splice sites by light blue boxes, and splicing patterns by diagonal lines joining the corresponding splice
sites. Loss-of-function mutations in the exon's coding sequence (black arrows) and mutations disrupting
the exon's flanking canonical splice sites (red arrows) usually affect the same transcriptional isoforms.

Comparison of phenotype variability

To compare phenotypes between probands, we computed the absolute difference in

scores (IQ, VABS, etc.) between pairs of individuals. We paired probands based on whether or

not they are affected by similar LGD mutations. Specifically, we compared pairs of probands: (1)

with LGD mutations in the same gene, (2) with mutations in the same gene and within 1000 bp, (3) with mutations in the same exon, and (4) with mutations in the same exon and of the same gender. For each group of paired comparisons, we estimate the phenotypic variability by calculating the average absolute difference in scores across all pairs. To estimate the statistical significance of differences in phenotypic variability, we then used one-tailed Mann-Whitney U tests to compare pairwise differences.

Chromosomal distance between mutations

We computed the distance in base pairs between a pair of mutations in the same gene by taking the absolute difference between their chromosomal positions. For deletion mutations that affect a genomic interval (i.e. deletion of multiple base pairs), we used the chromosomal coordinates that lead to the smallest distance between mutations. For example, the distance between a deletion and an upstream mutation was calculated based on the 5' coordinate of the deleted sequence, while the distance to a downstream mutation was calculated based on the 3' coordinate. Our results remained essentially unchanged when alternate distance metrics, such as interval midpoints or maximal distances, were used (results not shown).

Protein sequence analyses

To calculate the position of ASD mutations in protein sequence, we mapped genomic coordinates onto their respective protein-coding sequences. Gene annotation data, including both genomic coordinates and the corresponding coding sequence intervals, were obtained from the Ensembl database using the BioMart interface (biomart.org) [98]. Using primary amino acid sequences for each protein, we mapped each LGD mutation to a resulting premature stop codon in protein sequence We calculated (1) the distance between induced stop codons in amino acid sequence and (2) the fraction of protein sequence truncated by each premature stop codons. We then calculated the correlation between the fraction of protein sequence affected (truncated) and the corresponding proband phenotype. The analysis of correlations between relative amino acid positions and IQ phenotypes includes a small number of variants from X/Y chromosomes (~2% of all variants). Very similar results are obtained when these variants are excluded from the analyses.

Due to alternative splicing, the peptide distance between mutations can vary across transcript isoforms. In the analyses presented in the paper, we analyzed the mean peptide distance across all isoforms. However, we also used other definitions of distance, including: the maximal distance, the distance in the longest transcript isoform of the gene (or "canonical" isoform), or the median distance. Our results were consistent across different measures of peptide distance.

We performed a test in which we controlled for the peptide-sequence proximity of mutations in the same exon. To produce random pairs of mutations with peptide distances similar to those observed for mutations in the same exon, we used a rejection sampling approach. The motivation for this approach was that we were able to easily sample pairs of mutations in the same gene (by randomly choosing observed pairs of mutations). However, we wanted the peptide distances between mutations to match a distance distribution similar to the distances between mutations in the same exon.

Thus, we calculated two log-normal peptide distance distributions: a target distribution

$t(d)$ (mean: 1.89, SD: 0.55) describing the distribution of distances between mutations in the

same exon, and a sampling distribution $s(d)$ (mean: 2.50, SD: 0.54) describing the distribution

of distances between mutations in the same gene, but not necessarily the same exon. Then, for a

randomly selected pair of mutations sampled with replacement, we accepted it as a null

distribution sample with acceptance probability:

$$p(\text{accept}) = \frac{t(d)}{m \cdot s(d)} \qquad (11)$$

Where m is a constant that bounds the likelihood ratio between the distributions. The resulting

rejection sampling algorithm generates samples approximating the target distribution $t(d)$ using

proposals from the sampling distribution $s(d)$.

We then estimated the statistical significance of our results by comparing the observed

differences in IQ to those observed for distance-matched sets of mutations in the null

distribution.

Identifying protein domains affected by LGD mutations

To identify functional domains in proteins affected by LGD mutations, we downloaded

domain annotations from the Pfam database [91]. We matched Uniprot accession codes to

register premature truncating codons (introduced into genes by LGD mutations) onto each

annotated protein sequence (Figure 3.27). We then identified LGD mutations truncating the same

domain of a protein. In this analysis, we assumed that both complete loss and partial truncation

of a domain would result in loss of the domain's function.

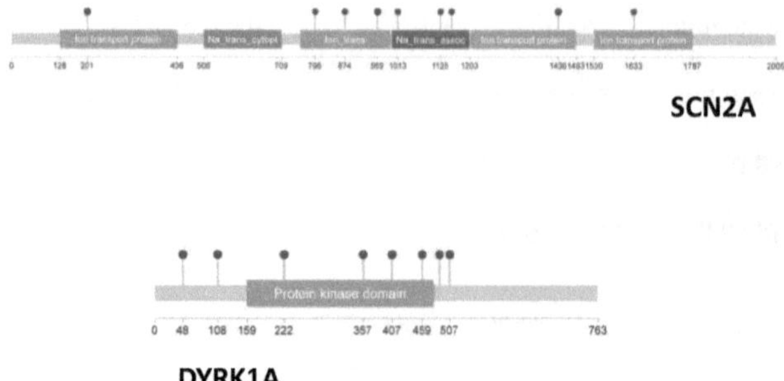

Figure 3.27 Illustration of mapping LGD mutations in SSC onto affected protein. Each bar diagram represents an example protein sequence (for SCN2A and DYRK1A), where subscript numbers represent coordinates in primary amino acid sequence. Colored boxes along the length of each sequence represent protein domains. Blue points represent LGD mutations in SSC mapped onto the corresponding protein sequence. Domains were identified using the Pfam database.

Enrichment of mutations in developmentally biased exons

For each exon in BrainSpan, we calculated the developmental bias statistic, defined as the difference between mean prenatal and mean postnatal expression levels. Means were calculated for log-transformed values ($\log_2 x+1$) across all prenatal or postnatal samples. Only exons expressed in the brain were considered (average RPKM $\geq$1). Exons from genes harboring LGD mutations were partitioned into quartile groups based on developmental bias. Enrichment in each exon group was calculated by comparing the fraction of LGD mutations affecting the grouped exons with the fraction of coding DNA sequences contained in the exons. Coding sequence lengths were obtained from Gencode v10 annotations.

In our analysis of GTEx data, we used our previously developed empirical Bayes model to calculate the percent of wild-type gene expression lost (Δx_{rel}) due to each LGD variant in GTEx. We then compared Δx_{rel} either between pairs of variants in the same exon or in the same gene but different exons.

Isoform-specific expression changes due to LGD variants

To quantify the effect of LGD variants on different splicing isoforms of a gene, we used our previously developed empirical Bayes model to calculate the change in expression separately for each transcriptional isoform of a gene. Importantly, we adapted our calculations to use RNA sequencing data summarized to isoform-specific expression levels. To that end, we introduced an indicator random variable (I), defined for each of k isoforms, which takes value 1 if an isoform contains the exon with the LGD mutation, and value 0 otherwise.

$$I_k = \begin{cases} 1 & \text{if isoform } k \text{ contains affected exon} \\ 0 & \text{otherwise} \end{cases} \tag{12}$$

To apply our model, we defined the observed expression level of the exon harboring an LGD mutation (x'_{exon} in Eqn. 2) as the sum of expression levels across all isoforms in a gene that are contain the affected exon, i.e.

$$x'_{\mathrm{exon}} = \sum_{\text{isoform } k} I_k x'_k \tag{13}$$

Where k indexes the isoforms of a gene and x'_k is the measured expression of the isoform. Then, analogous to our calculation for changes in the overall expression of a gene (see Eqn. 1), we calculated we calculated the change in expression of each isoform.

$$\Delta x_{\text{isoform } k} = \begin{cases} f \cdot \epsilon \cdot x_{\text{isoform } k} & \text{if isoform } k \text{ contains affected exon} \\ 0 & \text{otherwise} \end{cases} \qquad (14)$$

Which, using Equation 12, can be expressed more concisely as: $\Delta x_k = I_k \cdot f \cdot \epsilon \cdot x_k$.

To compare the effects of LGD mutations across n protein-coding isoforms of a gene, we represented the overall profile of all isoform expression changes as an n-dimensional vector:

$$\bar{z} = (\Delta x_{\text{isoform } 1}, \cdots, \Delta x_{\text{isoform } k}, \cdots, \Delta x_{\text{isoform } n}) \qquad (15)$$

To quantify the difference between isoform-specific expression change vectors, we used an angular distance metric between expression change vectors $\bar{z}_1$ and $\bar{z}_2$:

$$d(\bar{z}_1, \bar{z}_2) = \frac{2}{\pi} \cdot \cos^{-1} \frac{\bar{z}_1 \circ \bar{z}_2}{\|\bar{z}_1\|_2 \cdot \|\bar{z}_2\|_2} \qquad (16)$$

The dot ($\circ$) operator in the numerator represents the dot product between vectors. The denominator is the scalar product of the ℓ^2 (Euclidean) norms for each vector. In this way, the distance d, which takes values on the unit interval $[0,1]$, computes a normalized angle between the expression change vectors for LGD variants. As with total gene expression in the manuscript, we compared the distances d either between pairs of variants in the same exon or in the same gene but different exons.

4 Properties of exons and genes harboring LGD mutations in ASD

4.1 Introduction

Prior studies, including our previous work, analyzed important functional properties of genes with LGD mutations in ASD. For example, we and others identified common biological functions shared by target genes, expression biases towards specific cell types (including cortical neurons and striatal medium spiny neurons), and the widespread expression of ASD-associated genes throughout the human brain. These results have now been validated in multiple subsequent analyses. To our knowledge, however, no previous studies have investigated functional properties at the level of exons harboring autism-associated LGD mutations. Nor have previous studies connected functional properties of mutations, such as developmental expression or cell type-specific expression, to autism phenotypes in affected individuals. Building on previous work, we explored the functional properties of both target exons and genes and the relationships between such properties and ASD phenotypes.

Given the importance of exons in determining the phenotypic consequences of LGD mutations, in the presented studies we sought to characterize the expression-level properties of exons harboring LGD mutations in ASD. Specifically, we considered the expression level of target exons relative to other exons in the same gene, as well as changes in the expression of target exons across human development. We further investigated whether and to what extent probands' IQ phenotypes are associated with the identified patterns of exon expression.

We also performed a broad analysis of cell types in the brain that are likely to be affected by mutations in ASD. Specifically, we used recent large-scale single-cell sequencing datasets to implicate several novel cell types, including previously inaccessible neuronal populations and cells from novel brain regions. Based on these findings, we then considered possible correlations between mutations affecting implicated cell types and the phenotypic consequences observed in

affected probands. Finally, we investigated the relationship, in terms of phenotypic variance

explained, between changes in gene dosage, studied previously, and patterns of cell type-specific

expression.

4.2   Results

Given that relative exon usage varies across neural development [69, 99] and the strong association between exons and phenotypes, we explored how the developmental expression of exons relate to ASD phenotypes. To that end, we sorted exons from genes harboring LGD mutations [8] into four quartile groups based on their developmental expression bias, which was calculated as the fold-change between prenatal and postnatal exon expression levels (Figure 4.1a). We then analyzed the enrichment of LGD mutations in each exon group (see Methods). Compared to exons with no substantial developmental bias, we found significant enrichment of LGD mutations not only in exons with a strong prenatal bias (binomial one-tail test $p = 8 \times 10^3$, Relative Rate = 1.33), but also in exons with postnatal biases ($p = 0.018$, RR = 1.31) (Figure 4.1b).

To understand the phenotypes associated with these patterns of expression, we stratified probands into lower (≤ 70) and higher IQ (> 70) cohorts (Figure 4.1c). Interestingly, while LGD mutations associated with lower IQs were strongly enriched only in prenatally biased exons (binomial one-tail test $p = 6 \times 10^{-3}$, RR = 1.62), mutations associated with higher IQs were exclusively enriched in postnatally biased exons ($p = 0.05$, RR = 1.27). These results demonstrate that mutations in exons with biases towards prenatal and postnatal expression preferentially contribute to ASD cases with lower and higher IQ phenotypes, respectively. We note that the observed exon developmental biases for LGD mutations are not simply driven by biases at the gene level, as mutations associated with both higher and lower IQ phenotypes showed enrichment exclusively towards genes with prenatally biased expression (Figure 4.2).

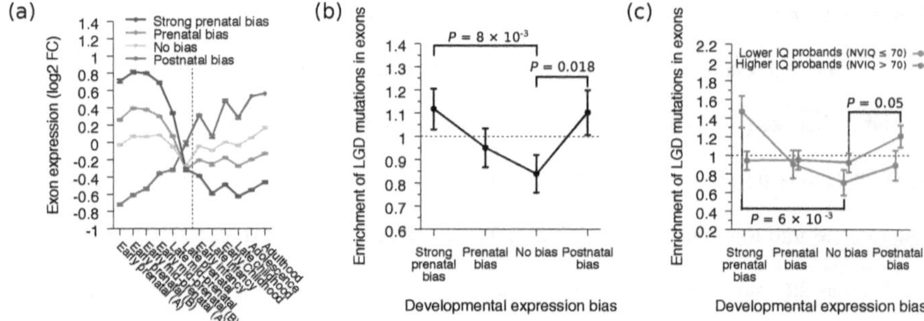

Figure 4.1 Relationship between the developmental expression of exons and intellectual ASD phenotypes. (a) Exon developmental expression profiles for genes with *de novo* LGD mutations in SSC. Exons from all genes harboring LGD mutations were sorted into four groups ("strong prenatal bias", "prenatal bias", "no bias", and "postnatal bias") based on their overall developmental expression bias; the developmental bias was calculated as the log₂ fold change between the average prenatal and postnatal exon expression levels. Lines represent the average expression profiles for exons in each group, and the x-axis represents 12 periods of human brain development, based on data from the Allen Institute's BrainSpan atlas [69]. The vertical dotted line delineates prenatal and postnatal developmental periods. Error bars represent the SEM. (b,c) Enrichment of LGD mutations across the four exon groups with different developmental biases. The y-axes represent the enrichment (relative rate) of mutations in each exon group; the enrichment was calculated by randomizing LGD mutations across exons proportionally to the exons' coding sequence lengths (see Methods). Error bars represent the SEM. (b) The overall enrichment of LGD mutations across the four exon groups of exons with different developmental expression biases. (c) The enrichment of LGD mutations across the four exon groups calculated separately for ASD probands with higher (>70, red) and lower (≤70, blue) nonverbal IQs.

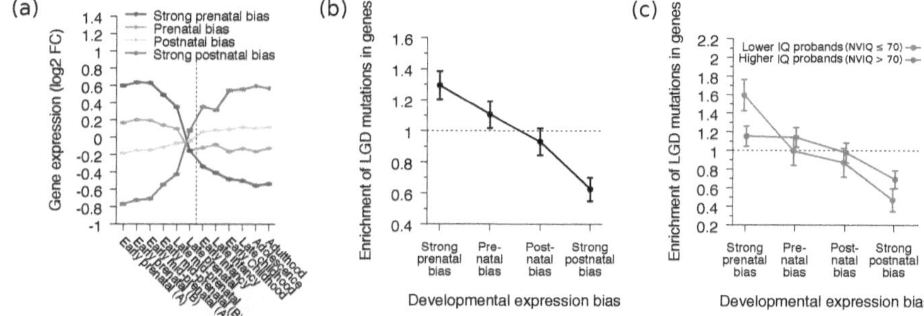

Figure 4.2 Relationship between the developmental expression profiles of ASD genes and IQ phenotypes. (a) Developmental expression profiles for genes harboring LGD mutations in SSC. Genes were grouped into four bins based on their developmental expression bias, i.e. the fold change between prenatal and postnatal expression. Lines represent the expression for genes in the four bins: genes with strong prenatal bias, genes with prenatal bias, genes with postnatal bias, and genes with strong postnatal bias. The x-axis represents different time periods across human brain development. The y-axis represents the relative expression of genes in each bin, defined as the average log2 fold-change relative to the mean expression level across all periods. Error bars represent the SEM. The vertical grey line delineates prenatal and postnatal developmental periods. (b,c) Enrichment of LGD mutations in genes across different bins (x-axis). The y-axes represent the enrichment of mutation in each group compared to the expected mutation frequency based on random shuffling of mutations across the full coding length of the corresponding protein. Error bars represent the SEM. (b) The enrichment of SSC LGD mutations in genes from the four bins. (c) The enrichment of SSC LGD mutations in the four bins for probands with higher (>70, red) and lower (<70, blue) nonverbal IQs.

Cell type-specific expression biases in ASD-associated genes

To understand which cell types are likely to be affected by mutations in ASD, we analyzed the expression of ASD genes in multiple cell type expression datasets. Initially, we used an expanded set of genes [100] to identify cell types expressing ASD genes at high levels. Specifically, we calculated the cell type-specific expression bias, defined as the difference, in standard deviations, between expression levels in a cell compared to the average expression level across all other cells (see Methods). By applying the approach to a commonly used TRAP-seq expression dataset [101, 102] of 24 genetically defined cell types in the mouse brain, we

99

identified biased expression towards multiple cell types, including deep layer projection neurons

in the cortex, inhibitory interneurons in the cortex, granule neurons in the cerebellum, and

medium spiny neurons in the striatum (Figure 4.3). Importantly, these findings both confirmed

and expanded on previous findings of ASD-associated cell types [5, 21, 103, 104].

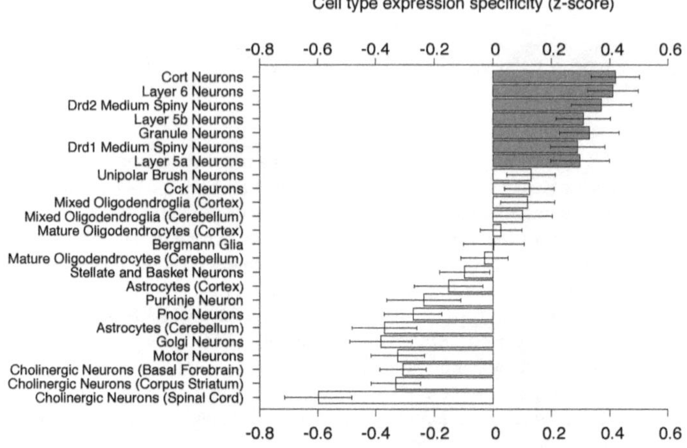

Figure 4.3 Cell type-specific expression biases in TRAP-seq dataset. Each bar represents the expression bias of ASD-associated genes towards a cell type. The x-axis represents the expression bias towards each cell type, calculated as the difference between the median specificity of ASD genes and the median specificity of genes with nonsynonymous mutations in siblings (see Methods). Along the y-axis, cell types are ordered by decreasing bias significance. Colored bars represent statistically significant biases (BH FDR $q \leq 0.05$), and empty bars represent biases that are not statistically significant. Error bars represent the SEM.

We also investigated the cell type expression biases in several single cell sequencing

datasets. One such dataset, the Harvard Brain Cell Atlas [105], comprised ~690,000 cells

collected from nine regions of the adult mouse brain. An analysis of 30 "metacell" clusters (i.e.

broad cell types based on unsupervised clustering) characterized in the dataset confirmed biases

towards neurons in the cortex (including pyramidal cells and inhibitory interneurons), striatum, and hippocampus, as well as novel cell populations in the amygdala and thalamus (Figure 4.4).

In an analysis of the Karolinka Institute's Mouse Brain Atlas [103, 106], which measured

expression in ~500,000 cells from 19 mouse brain regions and developmental periods, we

identified novel biases towards hippocampal neurons, serotonergic neurons, and developing cell

types including neuroblasts and embryonic neuronal populations (Figure 4.5). These results

suggest that many cell types in diverse regions of the brain may be affected in ASD.

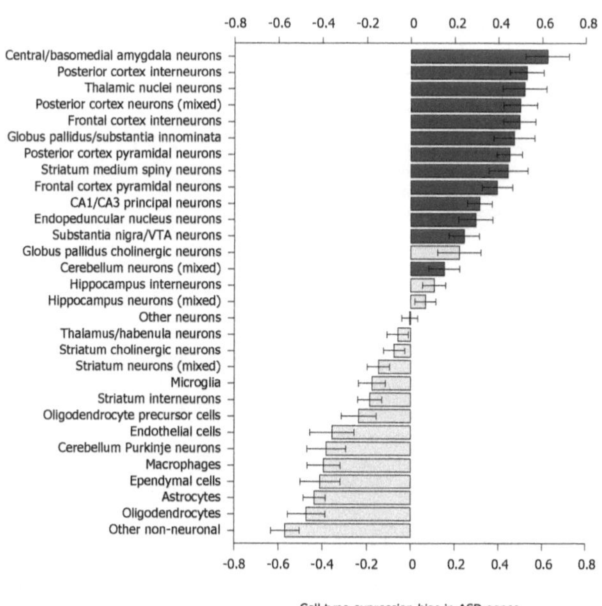

Figure 4.4 Cell type-specific expression biases in the Harvard Brain Cell Atlas. Each bar represents the expression bias of ASD-associated genes towards a cell type. The x-axis represents the expression bias towards each cell type, calculated as the difference between the median specificity of ASD genes and the median specificity of genes with nonsynonymous mutations in siblings (see Methods). Dark colored bars represent statistically significant biases (BH FDR $q \leq 0.05$), and light colored bars represent non-statistically significant biases. Error bars represent the SEM.

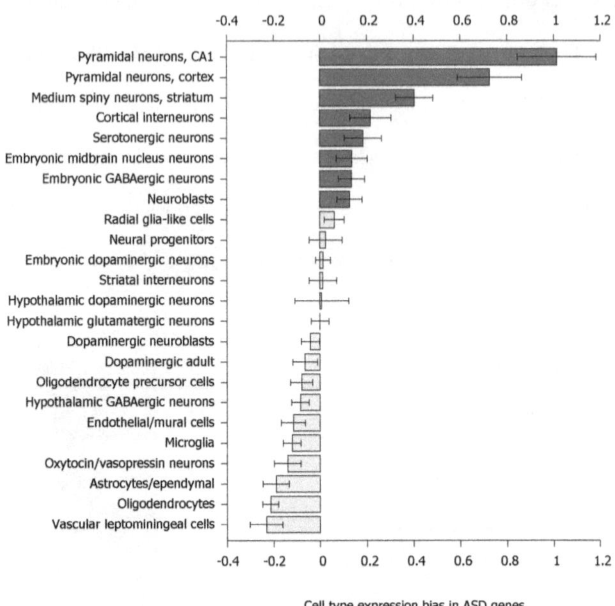

Figure 4.5 Cell type-specific expression biases in the Mouse Brain Atlas. Each bar represents the expression bias of ASD-associated genes towards a cell type. The x-axis represents the expression bias towards each cell type, calculated as the difference between the median specificity of ASD genes and the median specificity of genes with nonsynonymous mutations in siblings (see Methods). Dark colored bars represent statistically significant biases (BH FDR $q \leq 0.05$), and light colored bars represent non-statistically significant biases. Error bars represent the SEM.

We next investigated whether genes with different biological functions showed expression biases towards specific implicated cell types. To that end, we performed hierarchical cluster to identify functionally related ASD genes using a gene-gene interaction network [1, 5] (see Methods). Consistent with previous findings, we identified four functional clusters of genes: (1) chromatin modification genes, (2) transcription factors, (3) cytoskeletal and signaling genes, and (4) synaptic and ion-channel genes. Genes involved in chromatin modification and transcriptional regulation were, as expected, biased towards developing active neurons (Figure

4.6, blue). Interestingly, these developmentally active genes were also strongly biased towards

differentiated cell types in the adult brain, i.e. striatal, cortical, and hippocampal neurons.

Synaptic signaling and ion channel genes, on the other hand, were only biased towards adult

neurons (Figure 4.6, red).

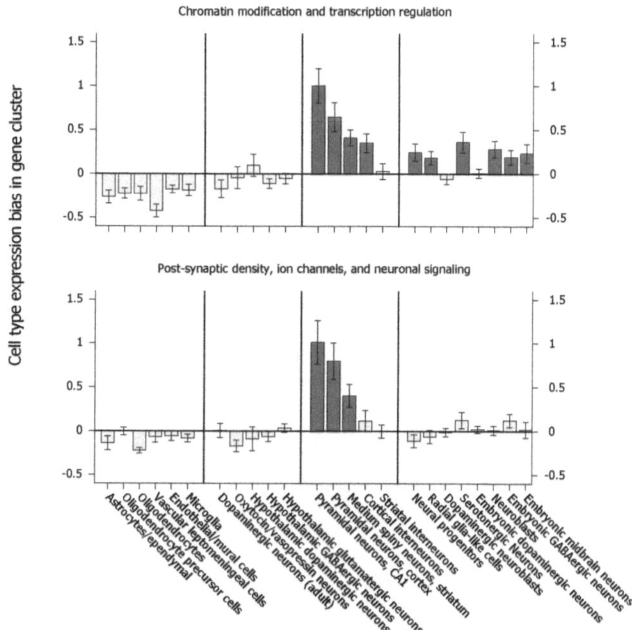

Figure 4.6 Cell type-specific expression biases grouped by biological function. Each bar represents the expression bias of ASD-associated genes towards a cell type. The y-axes represent expression biases towards cell type (see Methods). Panels represent the biases observed for genes in the chromatin modification and transcript factor clusters (top) or in the synaptic, signaling, and ion channel clusters (bottom). Dark colored bars represent statistically significant biases (BH FDR $q \leq 0.05$), and light colored bars represent biases that are not statistically significant. Error bars represent the SEM.

Interestingly, in addition to strong biases towards neurons, in general, and cortical

neurons, specifically, ASD-associated genes also showed biased expression between Drd1$^+$ (D1)

and Drd2$^+$ (D2) medium spiny neurons (MSN) in the striatum (Figure 4.7). On average, the biases towards D2 MSNs versus D1 MSNs, defined as the log₂ fold-change in expression, were

an order of magnitude larger for ASD genes than for genes with similar expression levels in

neurons; ASD mean bias = 0.12 versus expression-matched mean bias = 0.001; Wilcoxon rank-

sum on-tail test $p = 1.3 \times 10^{-7}$; statistical bootstrap $p \leq 1 \times 10^{-4}$. We then calculated, the enrichment

of D2 MSN-biased genes among ASD-associated genes. The analysis showed genes with

stronger biases towards D2 MSNs were also more enriched in ASD (Figure 4.8). Notably, these

expression biases between D2 and D1 MSNs, which have highly correlated gene expression

levels, suggests that mutations in ASD may have different functional effects even between

closely related cell types.

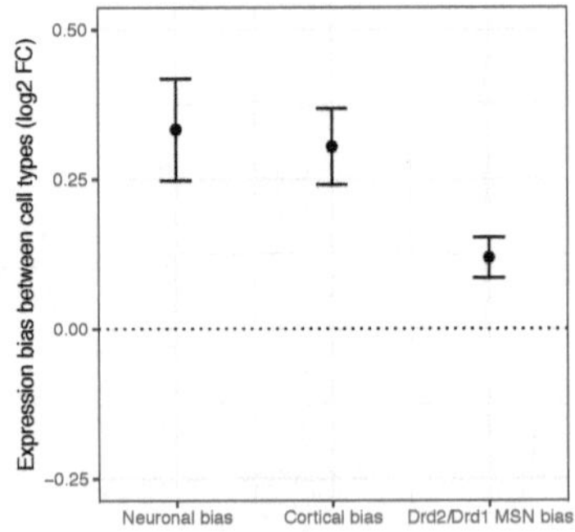

Figure 4.7 Comparative expression biases for ASD-associated genes. In each analysis, we compared expression biases between different cell populations in the mouse brain. From left to right along the x-axis, we considered bias differentials between neurons and non-neurons, cortical neurons and non-cortical neurons, and between Drd2+ and Drd1+ medium spiny neurons (MSN). The y-axis represents the average difference in bias for autism genes, normalized by the average difference for all genes. Standard errors were estimated by statistical bootstrapping. The dotted line represents values for no observable bias. Error bars represent the SEM.

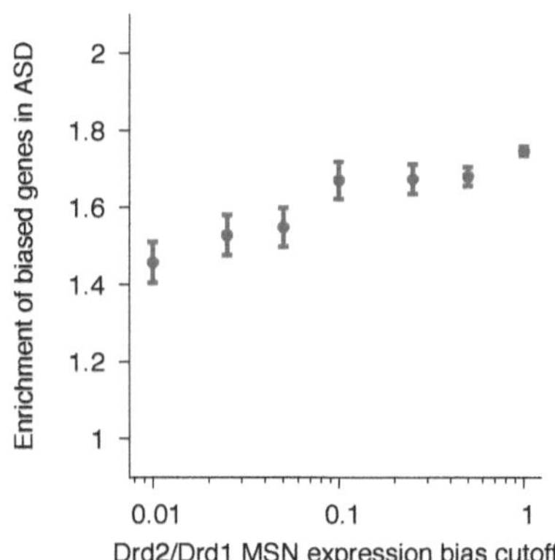

Figure 4.8 Enrichment of LGD mutations for genes with biased expression in MSNs. Genes were grouped by expression bias towards D2 versus D2 medium spiny neurons. Points represent the observed enrichment of bias-grouped genes among ASD-associated. The x-axis represents the minimum D2/D1 bias for the considered genes. The y-axis represents the enrichment of genes among ASD genes, i.e. the fraction of genes in each bias-group for ASD-genes normalized by the expected fraction. Expected fractions were estimated by randomizing genes proportional to their coding sequence lengths. Error bars represent the SEM.

Phenotypes associated with expression biases toward neuronal cell types

Given the diversity of cell types affected by ASD-associated mutations, we next

investigated whether mutations in genes biased towards different implicated cell types would

have different phenotypic consequences. To explore such relationships, we considered only

ASD-associated genes harboring likely gene-disrupting (LGD) mutations, which are likely to

have especially large phenotypic effects, in the Simons Simplex Collection (SSC) [8]. We then

compared the phenotype scores for individuals affected by LGD mutations with the expression

bias towards implicated cell types (see Methods). We found that expression biases towards

cortical neurons were significantly associated with the severity of specific ASD phenotypes,

including nonverbal IQ, social cognition, and adaptive behavior (Mann-Kendall trend test $p =$

105

0.031, 0.009, 0.026; Figure 4.9, left). Similarly, mutations affecting genes with expression biases towards cerebellar projection neurons (i.e. Purkinje cells, granule cells, and deep cerebellar nuclei) were associated with decreases in fine motor skills and general coordination (MK $p =$ 0.015, 0.033; Figure 4.9, right).

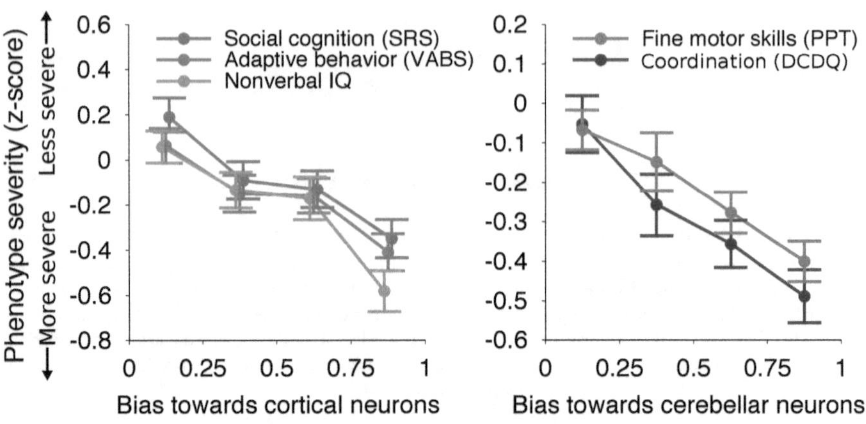

Figure 4.9 Association between cell type-specific expression and ASD phenotype severity. Each plot shows the severity of ASD phenotypes versus the specificity of genes towards specific cell types. Genes harboring LGD were grouped into four quartile bins based on their expression specificity towards (a) cortical neurons or (b) cerebellar projection neurons. The x-axes show the expression specificity quantiles for each bin. The y-axes show the standardized severity of (a) cognitive, adaptive, and social phenotypes or (b) fine motor skills and coordination phenotypes. Phenotypes were adjusted for age and gender, then normalized to z-scores (see Methods). Error bars represent the SEM.

Combined effects of dosage changes and cell-type specificity

Importantly, our previous analyses of cell type-to-phenotype relationships did not account for either dosage changes due to LGD variants or the sensitivity of phenotypes to changes in dosage (PDS). Since both are important determinants of the severity of phenotypes (see Chapter 2), we decided to use our previously developed models to investigate the phenotypic variance explained by both dosage and cell-type specificity. To generalize our analysis beyond individual scores and to reduce the number of hypotheses tested, we performed

PCA-based dimensional reduction (see Methods) on an expanded dataset of 31 phenotype scores.

The result of the procedure was three summary scores ("eigen-scores"), each a linear

combination of multiple raw scores, with each summary score representing a different axis of

autism phenotypes: (1) social and cognitive ability, (2) repetitive behaviors, and (3) motor skills.

These scores were only weakly correlated (Spearman's ρ = 0.26, 0.42, 0.24, for social-repetitive,

social-motor, and repetitive-motor, respectively).

To analyze the aforementioned scores, we initially applied our previously developed

PDS/dosage model, which accounts for phenotype severity due differences in effect on gene

dosage across exons as well as phenotype sensitivity to dosage changes of different genes.

Consistent with our previous findings, the normalized phenotypic effects for these aggregated

phenotypes were strongly correlated with relative exon expression (social/repetitive/motor

Pearson's R = 0.61, 0.44, 0.65; Figure 4.10). Interestingly, by correlating the PDS values for

phenotypes across genes, we observed that different phenotypes often had different sensitivities

to changes in the dosage of the same gene (Spearman's ρ = 0.22, 0.7, 0.45 for social-repetitive,

social-motor, and repetitive-motor). These results are to be expected, as genes can have very

different functions.

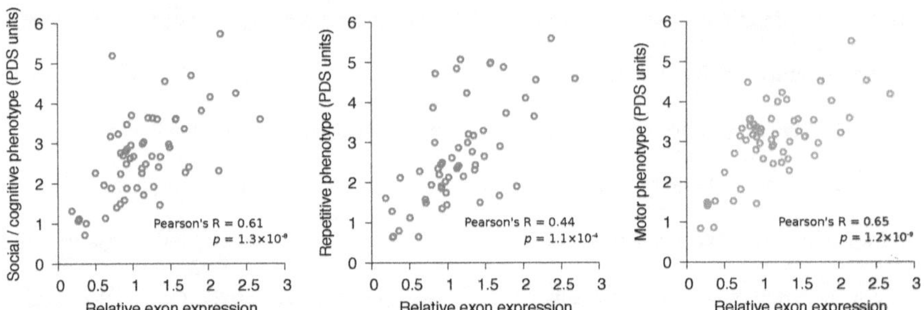

Figure 4.10 Correlation between relative exon expression and normalized phenotypic effects. Each point represents a proband with an LGD mutations in SSC. The x-axis represents the relative expression of the target exon, i.e. the exon expression level divided by the gene expression level. The y-axis represents the normalized effects of LGD mutations on aggregated (a) social and cognitive (b) repetitive and (c) motor skill phenotypes. Scores were normalized by the PDS values of target genes (see Methods).

Given that these models only explain part (~20-40%) of the phenotypic variance in ASD probands, we then considered whether the expression biases towards specific cell types could explain additional phenotypic variability not captured by PDS/dosage models. To investigate, we used our dosage models to normalize phenotypes, as described above. We then fitted a least-squares linear regression between the relative exon expression and normalized phenotype scores, and used the residuals – i.e. the normalized variance unexplained by the model – as phenotype scores. Importantly, the procedure allowed us to investigate whether cell type-specific expression affects phenotypes after account for variance due to differences in gene dosage.

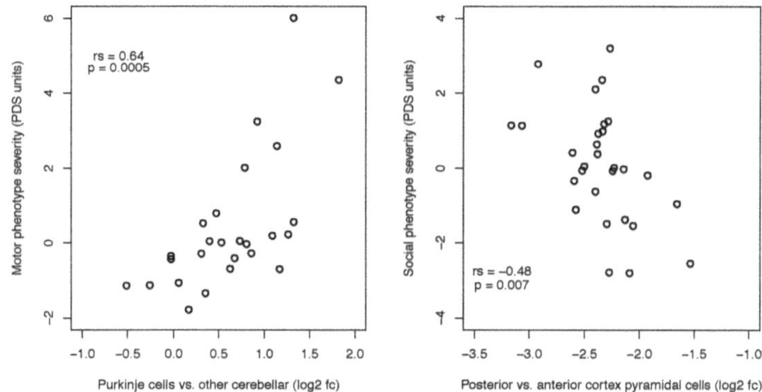

Figure 4.11 Residual phenotypic variance explained by pairwise cell type expression biases. Each point in scatterplots represents a proband affected by an LGD mutation in SSC. The x-axis represents the expression bias of the target gene. Biases were calculated as the fold-change between (a) Purkinje cells and other cerebellar cells or between (b) pyramidal cells in the posterior and anterior cortex. The y-axis represents the residual phenotype severity (i.e. severity after normalizing for gene dosage and PDS) for (a) motor skills or (b) social phenotypes.

To model the residual phenotypes, we calculated the rank correlations between cell type expression biases and the residual phenotype scores (Figure 4.11). As explanatory variables, we calculated pairwise biases in expression between related cell types. Specifically, we performed hierarchical clustering to identify related cell types. Then for each merge in the clustering tree, we calculated the gene expression biases (i.e. difference in specificity) between merged cell types. Interestingly, we found that differences in expression indeed explain a substantial fraction of the variance. The expression between Purkinje cells and granule cells in the cerebellum, for example, correlated strongly with residual motor phenotypes (Spearman's $\rho = 0.64$, Benjamini-Hochberg FDR $q = 0.0005$). We also found that expression biases towards the posterior cortex, versus anterior cortex, were inversely correlated with the residual severity of social phenotypes ($\rho = -0.48$, BH FDR $q = 0.007$). These results suggest that differences in expression between cell populations correlate with phenotype severity, explaining ~40% and ~25% of the residual phenotypic variance. Importantly, these relationships are independent of the relationship between dosage and phenotypes. Cumulatively, these relatively simple models of phenotypes likely explain ~50-65% of the variance across individual probands.

4.3 Methods

To calculate the developmental expression biases, we used expression data from the
BrainSpan expression atlas [69]. For the analysis, we used RNA-seq Gencode v10 summarized
data, available online (http://brainspan.org/static/download.html). Expression values were log-
scaled and domain-shifted by a pseudocount ($\log_2 x+1$). Means were calculated across all
prenatal or postnatal samples. Only exons expressed in the brain were considered (average
RPKM ≥ 1). The developmental expression bias was calculated as the log fold-change (i.e. the
difference in log-scale) between the average prenatal and postnatal expression levels.

To calculate enrichment in exon groups, all exons from genes harboring LGD mutations
were partitioned into quartile groups based on developmental bias. Enrichments in each exon
group were calculated by comparing the fraction of LGD mutations affecting the exons with
fraction of coding sequence in the exons' coding sequences (CDS). Coding sequence lengths
were obtained from Gencode v10 annotations. Relative rates reported for developmentally biased
exon groups were calculated by comparing the enrichment in the biased group to the enrichment
observed for exons with no developmental bias.

Single cell-type specific expression data was obtained from multiple ongoing projects.
From the Karolinska Institute's Mouse Brain Atlas, we analyzed single-cell expression data
~500,000 cells from 19 regions of the developing and adult mouse brain [106]. Specifically, we
downloaded a commonly used prepared dataset summarized expression to 24 cell type clusters
avalailable online (http://mousebrain.org/downloads.html). From the Harvard Brain Cell Atlas,

111

we obtained data for ~690,000 cells from nine regions of the adult mouse brain, which had been

clustered into 30 broad cell-type classes (aggregated metacell dataset; http://dropviz.org/) [107].

Finally, we applied our developed methods to a previously analyzed dataset of 24 cell types with

expression levels characterized using TRAP-seq [101, 102]. To analyze ASD genes using cell

type expression datasets from the mouse brain, we mapped human genes onto mouse orthologs

using the NCBI Homologene database [108].

To analyze the aforementioned datasets, we calculated the specificity of genes towards

each cell type. Specifically, for each cell type, we defined the specificity bias of expression as

the difference from the mean across all cell types in standard deviations, i.e.

$$z_c = \frac{x_c - \mu_X}{\sigma_X}$$

Where z_c represents the expression specificity towards cell type c, x_c represents the expression

level of the gene in that cell type, μ_X represents the average expression across all cell types, and

σ_X represents the standard deviation of expression across all cells. The reported ASD bias

statistics for each cell type were calculated as the difference between median specificity for

ASD-associated genes and median specificity for genes with nonsynonymous mutations in

unaffected siblings ($\tilde{z}_{ASD} - \tilde{z}_{\text{sibling}}$). Significance was tested using a Mann-Whitney U one-tail

test and adjusted for multiple hypotheses with a Benjamini-Hochberg FDR correction.

Grouping ASD-associated genes by biological function

To group ASD-associated genes by biological function, we adapted a method developed

in our previous work. Specifically, we used a gene-gene interaction network (i.e. NETBAG+),

where edged between genes represented the probability of genes contributing to similar biological function. We used an updated version of the network (available by request) to perform

the clustering.

Using the gene-gene interaction network, we calculated the similarity between genes as

the Spearman rank correlation between interactions across all other genes in the network. We

converted similarity measures to distance measures by calculating 1-ρ, where ρ represents the

calculated rank correlation. We then used agglomerative hierarchical clustering with Ward's

linkage criterion to group genes. Based on previous findings, we divided genes into four clusters,

namely chromatin modification, transcription factors, cytoskeleton and signaling, and synaptic

genes. We then analyzed cell-type specific biases for each functional cluster of genes.

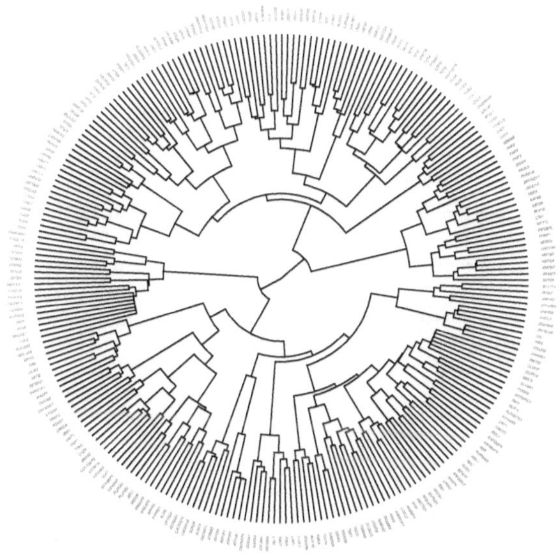

Figure 4.12 Radial dendrogram of functional clusters of ASD genes. ASD-associated genes were hierarchically clustered based on pairwise similarity (1-correlation) of edge weights on a gene-gene interaction network (see Methods). Clustering was done using Ward's linkage criterion. Gene labels were colored by functional group.

In the analyses of autism phenotype scores, we considered SSC probands, notably of different genders and spanning a broad range of ages. To account for developmental differences across age and gender, for each phenotype statistically significantly (FDR ≤ 0.05) correlated with age or gender, we adjusted phenotypic scores to account for these variables. We used a binary variable (taking value 0 for male or 1 for female) to estimate significant mean differences across genders. Following a previously developed approach [97], we adjusted scores using linear regression. Specifically, we performed a multivariate linear regression for each phenotypic score, with age and/or gender as independent regression parameters. We then used the regression residuals as adjusted scores for comparing proband phenotypes. We approximated probands' ages as the age at which Autism Diagnostic Observation Schedule was administered (i.e. "age at ADOS").

After regression, we standardized scores to phenotypic z-scores, defined as the difference, in standard deviations, between a given proband's phenotype score and the average score across all probands. The procedure centered and scaled phenotypic scores for combined analysis of multiple phenotypes.

To study the effects across a larger set of phenotype scores, we performed dimensional reduction to summarize phenotypes. Specifically, we used a defined list of scores available in SSC, which were curated by SSC clinicians to capture important phenotypic features of autism ("Core Descriptive Variables" in the Phenotype Data Dictionary). These scores were further grouped into several phenotype categories, with groups of scores quantifying adaptive/cognitive, language/communication, social, and repetitive behaviors. We used SSC Version 15, Phenotype Data Set 9, available on SFARI Base.

For each group of core descriptive variables, we performed Principal Component Analysis (PCA), after centering and scaling variables. We then considered the first principle component (PC), i.e. the linear combination of scores explaining the most inter-individual variance for all scores in the group, and used it as a summary score for the represented behavior. Importantly, for each group, these principal components explained a majority of the total variance (~45-80%, Figure 4.13) suggesting that our method effectively captures the phenotypic variation in common between all scores. Component directions were chosen so that higher scores represent more severe phenotypes.

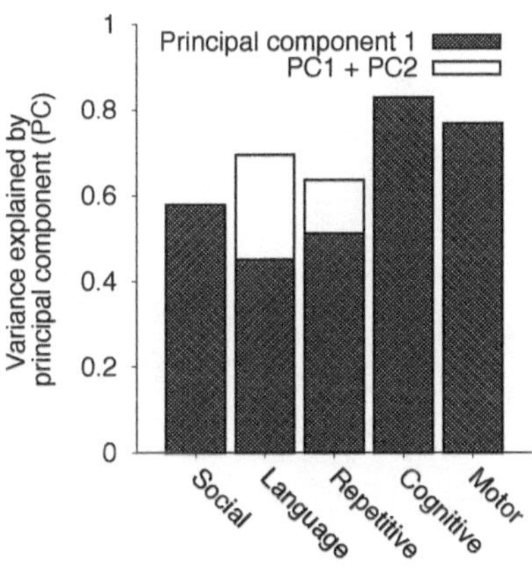

Figure 4.13 Variance explained by eigenphenotypes. Principal components were calculated for each set of curated phenotypes in SSC. From left to right, the x-axis represents social, language, repetitive, cognitive, and motor skill phenotype scores. The y-axis represents the variance explained by either the first principal component (colored bars) or cumulatively by both the first and second principal components (light bars).

Although our approach reduced the dimensionality of the phenotype dataset, it did not guarantee either independence or zero correlations between phenotypes. Consequently, we calculated the correlations between all pairs of scores (Figure 4.14). Based on the analysis, we further grouped the social, language, and cognitive phenotype groups. We then performed PCA to obtain a summary score for the combined group of scores.

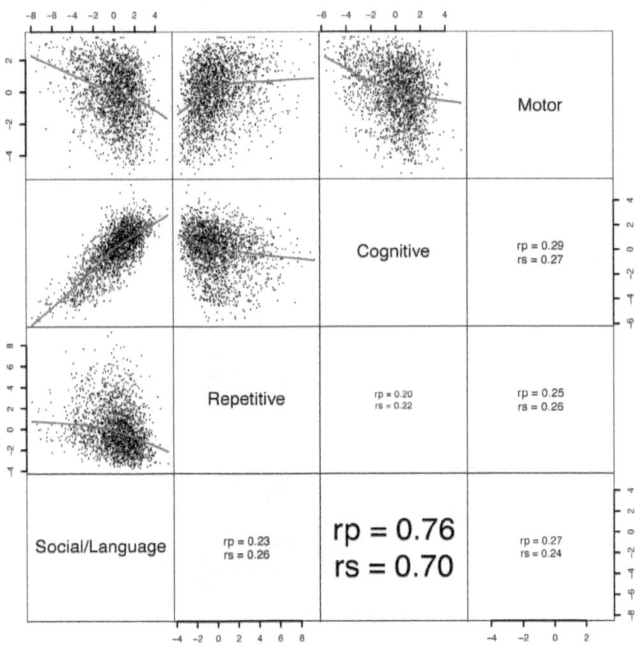

Figure 4.14 Correlation between aggregated phenotypes. In the upper triangle of the grid: Each point in the scatterplots represents a proband in SSC. The x-axes represent scores for the aggregated phenotype in the text label below the scatterplot. The y-axes represent scores for the aggregated phenotype labeled to the right of the scatterplot. Red lines represent spline regressions between variables. In the lower triangle of the grid: Each box represents the Pearson (rp) or Spearman (rs) correlation, calculated across all probands, between aggregated phenotype scores. For each box, the correlated phenotypes are labeled along the diagonal to the left and above. The size of correlation coefficients is proportional to the strength of the correlation.

Conclusion

Previous studies explored phenotypic similarity in syndromic forms of ASD due to mutations in specific genes [51, 54, 56, 109, 110]. Nevertheless, across a large collection of contributing genes, the nature of the substantial phenotypic heterogeneity in ASD is not well understood. Interestingly, the diversity of intellectual and other important ASD phenotypes resulting from *de novo* LGD mutations in the same genes is usually only slightly (~10%) smaller than the phenotypic diversity across the entire ASD cohort. The presented studies explored multiple biological mechanisms contributing to phenotypic heterogeneity in simplex ASD cases triggered by LGD mutations.

Truncating mutations, even in the same gene, can have different NMD-mediated effects on gene dosage. Heterozygous truncating genotypes on average decrease gene expression by ~15-30%, but effect sizes vary across several orders of magnitude. Such differences in the dosage effects of truncating mutations likely contribute to the phenotypic variability across probands. In addition to effects associated with different changes in gene dosage, there is also substantial variability in the sensitivity of a phenotype to changes in the dosage of specific genes. When dosage-sensitivities are taken into account (for example, using gene-specific PDS values), predicted dosage changes correlate strongly with the severity of phenotypes ($R^2 \sim 0.4$). These quantitative relationship between changes in dosage and phenotype are likely to specific phenotype-gene pairs.

Perturbations leading to similar dosage changes in the same gene may affect different, functionally distinct splicing isoforms. However, when exactly the same sets of isoforms are perturbed, as for LGD mutations in the same exon, the resulting phenotypes, even in unrelated ASD probands, are especially similar. For LGD mutations affecting intellectual phenotypes, we found that same exon membership accounts for a larger fraction of phenotypic variance than multiple other genomic features, including expression, evolutionary conservation, pathway membership, and domain truncation. There are likely deviations from these patterns for specific genes and specific mutations. For example, truncated proteins that escape NMD may lead to partial buffering, due to remaining activity, or to further damaging effects, due to dominant negative interactions. Nevertheless, our results suggest that for *de novo* LGD mutations in ASD, exons, rather than genes, often represent a unit of effective phenotypic impact.

The dosage models developed in the present work can likely be applied in other contexts. While we studied dosage changes due to NMD of truncating variants, other mechanisms of dosage change, such as regulatory mutations, may also be used to characterize dosage-trait relationships. As genetic and phenotypic data accumulate, it will be interesting to estimate the sensitivity of multiple phenotypes for a substantial number of ASD risk genes. Furthermore, given the consistent patterns of gene and isoform-specific dosage effects across tissues, it may be possible to estimate sensitivity parameters (i.e. PDS) for other genetic disorders and phenotypes. In this respect, quantitative gene-dosage relationships have been recently characterized for yeast fitness values in different environmental conditions [111].

The present study focused specifically on simplex cases of ASD, in which *de novo* LGD mutations are highly penetrant and where the contribution of genetic background is minimized. It is likely that differences in genetic background and environment represent other important sources of phenotypic variability [22, 61, 112]. Therefore, in more diverse cohorts, individuals with LGD mutations in the same exon will likely display greater phenotypic heterogeneity. For example, the Simons Variation in Individuals Project has identified broad spectra of phenotypes associated with specific variants in more general populations [29, 113-115]. Similarly, probands from trio families (i.e. with no unaffected siblings) show greater variability in phenotypes. For these probands, the enrichment of *de novo* LGD mutations is substantially lower and the contribution from genetic background is likely to be larger [34], resulting in more pronounced phenotypic variability.

Our study may have important implications for precision medicine [112, 116, 117]. The presented results indicate that relatively mild decreases in gene dosage may account for a substantial fraction of adverse phenotypic consequences. Thus, from a therapeutic perspective, compensatory expression of intact alleles, as demonstrated in mouse models of ASD [118-120] and other diseases [121], may provide an approach for alleviating phenotypic effects for at least a fraction of ASD cases. From a prognostic perspective, our results suggest that by sequencing and phenotyping sufficiently large patient cohorts with truncating mutations in different exons, it may be possible to understand likely phenotypic consequences originating from LGD mutations in specific exons. Furthermore, because we observed consistent patterns of expression changes across multiple human tissues, similar analyses may be also extended to other disorders affected by highly penetrant truncating mutations.

References

1.   Gilman, S.R., et al., *Diverse types of genetic variation converge on functional gene networks involved in schizophrenia.* Nature Neuroscience, 2012. **15**(12): p. 1723-8.

2.   Ayalew, M., et al., *Convergent functional genomics of schizophrenia: from comprehensive understanding to genetic risk prediction.* Molecular Psychiatry, 2012. **17**(9): p. 887-905.

3.   Fromer, M., et al., *De novo mutations in schizophrenia implicate synaptic networks.* Nature, 2014. **506**(7487): p. 179-184.

4.   Parikshak, N.N., M.J. Gandal, and D.H. Geschwind, *Systems biology and gene networks in neurodevelopmental and neurodegenerative disorders.* Nature Reviews Genetics, 2015. **16**(8): p. 441-458.

5.   Chang, J., et al., *Genotype to phenotype relationships in autism spectrum disorders.* Nature Neuroscience, 2015. **18**(2): p. 191-198.

6.   Gilman, S.R., et al., *Rare de novo variants associated with autism implicate a large functional network of genes involved in formation and function of synapses.* Neuron, 2011. **70**(5): p. 898-907.

7.   Sanders, S.J., et al., *Multiple recurrent de novo CNVs, including duplications of the 7q11.23 Williams syndrome region, are strongly associated with autism.* Neuron, 2011. **70**(5): p. 863-85.

8.   Iossifov, I., et al., *The contribution of de novo coding mutations to autism spectrum disorder.* Nature, 2014. **515**(7526): p. 216-21.

9.   Satterstrom, F.K., et al., *Large-Scale Exome Sequencing Study Implicates Both Developmental and Functional Changes in the Neurobiology of Autism.* Cell, 2020.

10.   O'Roak, B.J., et al., *Sporadic autism exomes reveal a highly interconnected protein network of de novo mutations.* Nature, 2012. **485**(7397): p. 246-50.

11.   American Psychiatric Association (DSM-5 Task Force), *Diagnostic and Statistical Manual of Mental Disorders: DSM-5.* 5th ed. 2013, Washington, DC: American Psychiatric Association.

12.   Krumm, N., et al., *A de novo convergence of autism genetics and molecular neuroscience.* Trends in Neuroscience, 2014. **37**(2): p. 95-105.

13.   Ronemus, M., et al., *The role of de novo mutations in the genetics of autism spectrum disorders.* Nature Reviews Genetics, 2014. **15**(2): p. 133-41.

14.   de la Torre-Ubieta, L., et al., *Advancing the understanding of autism disease mechanisms through genetics.* Nat Med, 2016. **22**(4): p. 345-61.

15.   Jeste, S.S. and D.H. Geschwind, *Disentangling the heterogeneity of autism spectrum disorder through genetic findings.* Nature Reviews Neurology, 2014. **10**(2): p. 74-81.

16.   Talkowski, M.E., E.V. Minikel, and J.F. Gusella, *Autism Spectrum Disorder Genetics: Diverse Genes with Diverse Clinical Outcomes.* Harvard Review of Psychiatry, 2014. **22**(2): p. 65-75.

17.   Gaugler, T., et al., *Most genetic risk for autism resides with common variation.* Nature Genetics, 2014. **46**(8): p. 881-5.

18.   Gratten, J., et al., *Large-scale genomics unveils the genetic architecture of psychiatric disorders.* Nature Neuroscience, 2014. **17**(6): p. 782-90.

19.   Anney, R., et al., *Individual common variants exert weak effects on the risk for autism spectrum disorders.* Human Molecular Genetics, 2012. **21**(21): p. 4781-4792.

20.   Krumm, N., et al., *Excess of rare, inherited truncating mutations in autism.* Nature Genetics, 2015. **47**(6): p. 582-8.

21.   Turner, T.N., et al., *Genomic Patterns of De Novo Mutation in Simplex Autism.* Cell, 2017. **171**(3): p. 710-722.e12.

22.   Robinson, E.B., et al., *Autism spectrum disorder severity reflects the average contribution of de novo and familial influences.* Proceedings of the National Academy of Sciences, 2014. **111**(42): p. 15161-15165.

23.   Levy, D., et al., *Rare de novo and transmitted copy-number variation in autistic spectrum disorders.* Neuron, 2011. **70**(5): p. 886-97.

24.   Buja, A., et al., *Damaging de novo mutations diminish motor skills in children on the autism spectrum.* Proceedings of the National Academy of Sciences, 2018. **115**(8): p. E1859-E1866.

25.   Taylor, L.J., et al., *Are there differences in the behavioural phenotypes of Autism Spectrum Disorder probands from simplex and multiplex families?* Research in Autism Spectrum Disorders, 2015. **11**: p. 56-62.

26.	Dissanayake, C., et al., *Cognitive and behavioral differences in toddlers with autism spectrum disorder from multiplex and simplex families.* Autism Research, 2019. **12**(4): p. 682-693.

27.	Berends, D., C. Dissanayake, and L.P. Lawson, *Differences in Cognition and Behaviour in Multiplex and Simplex Autism: Does Prior Experience Raising a Child with Autism Matter?* Journal of Autism and Developmental Disorders, 2019. **49**(8): p. 3401-3411.

28.	Fischbach, G.D. and C. Lord, *The Simons Simplex Collection: a resource for identification of autism genetic risk factors.* Neuron, 2010. **68**(2): p. 192-5.

29.	Simons VIP Consortium, *Simons Variation in Individuals Project (Simons VIP): a genetics-first approach to studying autism spectrum and related neurodevelopmental disorders.* Neuron, 2012. **73**(6): p. 1063-7.

30.	American Psychiatric Association DSM-5 Task Force, *Diagnostic and Statistical Manual of Mental Disorders: DSM-5.* 5th ed. 2013, Washington, DC: American Psychiatric Association.

31.	Baio, J., et al., *Prevalence of Autism Spectrum Disorder Among Children Aged 8 Years - Autism and Developmental Disabilities Monitoring Network, 11 Sites, United States, 2014.* MMWR Surveillance Summit, 2018. **67**(6): p. 1-23.

32.	Bourgeron, T., *From the genetic architecture to synaptic plasticity in autism spectrum disorder.* Nature Reviews Neuroscience, 2015. **16**(9): p. 551-563.

33.	Sandin, S., et al., *The Heritability of Autism Spectrum Disorder.* JAMA, 2017. **318**(12): p. 1182-1184.

34.	Zhao, X., et al., *A unified genetic theory for sporadic and inherited autism.* Proceedings of the National Academy of Sciences, 2007. **104**(31): p. 12831-12836.

35.	O'Roak, B.J., et al., *Sporadic autism exomes reveal a highly interconnected protein network of de novo mutations.* Nature, 2012. **485**: p. 246-246.

36.	Iossifov, I., et al., *De novo gene disruptions in children on the autistic spectrum.* Neuron, 2012. **74**(2): p. 285-99.

37.	Yuen, R.K.C., et al., *Whole genome sequencing resource identifies 18 new candidate genes for autism spectrum disorder.* Nature Neuroscience, 2017. **20**: p. 602-611.

38.	Anney, R.J.L., et al., *Meta-analysis of GWAS of over 16,000 individuals with autism spectrum disorder highlights a novel locus at 10q24.32 and a significant overlap with schizophrenia.* Molecular Autism, 2017. **8**(1): p. 21.

39.   Lord, C., et al., *Autism spectrum disorder.* Nature Reviews Disease Primers, 2020. **6**(1): p. 5.

40.   De Rubeis, S., et al., *Synaptic, transcriptional and chromatin genes disrupted in autism.* Nature, 2014. **515**(7526): p. 209-215.

41.   Chang, J., et al., *Genotype to phenotype relationships in autism spectrum disorders.* Nature Neuroscience, 2015. **18**(2): p. 191-8.

42.   Parikshak, Neelroop N., et al., *Integrative Functional Genomic Analyses Implicate Specific Molecular Pathways and Circuits in Autism.* Cell, 2013. **155**(5): p. 1008-1021.

43.   Neale, B.M., et al., *Patterns and rates of exonic de novo mutations in autism spectrum disorders.* Nature, 2012. **485**: p. 242.

44.   Arguello, P.A. and J.A. Gogos, *Genetic and cognitive windows into circuit mechanisms of psychiatric disease.* Trends in Neurosciences, 2012. **35**(1): p. 3-13.

45.   Gordon, J.A., et al., *Challenges and Opportunities in Psychiatric Neuroscience.* Cold Spring Harbor Symposia on Quantitative Biology, 2018. **83**: p. 1-8.

46.   Bishop, S.L., et al., *Identification of Developmental and Behavioral Markers Associated with Genetic Abnormalities in Autism Spectrum Disorder.* The American Journal of Psychiatry, 2017. **174**(6): p. 576-585.

47.   Doshi-Velez, F., Y. Ge, and I. Kohane, *Comorbidity Clusters in Autism Spectrum Disorders: An Electronic Health Record Time-Series Analysis.* Pediatrics, 2014. **133**(1): p. e54.

48.   Chaste, P., et al., *A genome-wide association study of autism using the Simons Simplex Collection: Does reducing phenotypic heterogeneity in autism increase genetic homogeneity?* Biol Psychiatry, 2015. **77**(9): p. 775-84.

49.   Chen, J.A., et al., *The emerging picture of autism spectrum disorder: genetics and pathology.* Annu Rev Pathol, 2015. **10**: p. 111-44.

50.   Boyle, E.A., Y.I. Li, and J.K. Pritchard, *An Expanded View of Complex Traits: From Polygenic to Omnigenic.* Cell, 2017. **169**(7): p. 1177-1186.

51.   Sztainberg, Y. and H.Y. Zoghbi, *Lessons learned from studying syndromic autism spectrum disorders.* Nat Neurosci, 2016. **19**(11): p. 1408-1417.

52.   Zhang, F., et al., *Copy number variation in human health, disease, and evolution.* Annu Rev Genomics Hum Genet, 2009. **10**: p. 451-81.

53.   Leppa, V.M., et al., *Rare Inherited and De Novo CNVs Reveal Complex Contributions to ASD Risk in Multiplex Families.* Am J Hum Genet, 2016. **99**(3): p. 540-554.

54.   Bernier, R., et al., *Disruptive CHD8 mutations define a subtype of autism early in development.* Cell, 2014. **158**(2): p. 263-276.

55.   Earl, R.K., et al., *Clinical phenotype of ASD-associated DYRK1A haploinsufficiency.* Molecular Autism, 2017. **8**(1): p. 54.

56.   Van Bon, B., et al., *Disruptive de novo mutations of DYRK1A lead to a syndromic form of autism and ID.* Molecular Psychiatry, 2016. **21**(1): p. 126-132.

57.   Liu, Z., et al., *Autism-like behaviours and germline transmission in transgenic monkeys overexpressing MeCP2.* Nature, 2016. **530**(7588): p. 98-102.

58.   Sztainberg, Y., et al., *Reversal of phenotypes in MECP2 duplication mice using genetic rescue or antisense oligonucleotides.* Nature, 2015. **528**: p. 123.

59.   D'Angelo, D., et al., *Defining the Effect of the 16p11.2 Duplication on Cognition, Behavior, and Medical Comorbidities.* JAMA Psychiatry, 2016. **73**(1): p. 20-30.

60.   Huguet, G., E. Ey, and T. Bourgeron, *The Genetic Landscapes of Autism Spectrum Disorders.* Annual Review of Genomics and Human Genetics, 2013. **14**(1): p. 191-213.

61.   Robinson, E.B., et al., *Genetic risk for autism spectrum disorders and neuropsychiatric variation in the general population.* Nature Genetics, 2016. **48**(5): p. 552-555.

62.   Fischbach, G.D. and C. Lord, *The Simons Simplex Collection: A Resource for Identification of Autism Genetic Risk Factors.* Neuron, 2010. **68**(2): p. 192-195.

63.   Ronemus, M., et al., *The role of de novo mutations in the genetics of autism spectrum disorders.* Nature Reviews Genetics, 2014. **15**: p. 133.

64.   Chang, Y.F., J.S. Imam, and M.F. Wilkinson, *The nonsense-mediated decay RNA surveillance pathway.* Annu Rev Biochem, 2007. **76**: p. 51-74.

65.   Rivas, M.A., et al., *Human genomics. Effect of predicted protein-truncating genetic variants on the human transcriptome.* Science, 2015. **348**(6235): p. 666-9.

66.   Melé, M., et al., *The human transcriptome across tissues and individuals.* Science, 2015. **348**(6235): p. 660.

67.   Findlay, G.M., et al., *Saturation editing of genomic regions by multiplex homology-directed repair.* Nature, 2014. **513**(7516): p. 120-123.

68.   Blomen, V.A., et al., *Gene essentiality and synthetic lethality in haploid human cells.* Science, 2015: p. aac7557.

69.   Kang, H.J., et al., *Spatio-temporal transcriptome of the human brain.* Nature, 2011. **478**(7370): p. 483-489.

70.   Nagy, E. and L.E. Maquat, *A rule for termination-codon position within intron-containing genes: when nonsense affects RNA abundance.* Trends in Biochemical Sciences, 1998. **23**(6): p. 198-199.

71.   Haworth, C.M.A., et al., *The heritability of general cognitive ability increases linearly from childhood to young adulthood.* Molecular Psychiatry, 2009. **15**(11): p. 1112-1120.

72.   Sparrow, S.S., et al., *Vineland adaptive behavior scales : interview edition, survey form manual.* 1984, Circle Pines, Minn.: American Guidance Service.

73.   Sanders, S.J., et al., *De novo mutations revealed by whole-exome sequencing are strongly associated with autism.* Nature, 2012. **485**(7397): p. 237-41.

74.   O'Roak, B.J., et al., *Exome sequencing in sporadic autism spectrum disorders identifies severe de novo mutations.* Nat Genet, 2011. **43**(6): p. 585-9.

75.   McLaren, W., et al., *Deriving the consequences of genomic variants with the Ensembl API and SNP Effect Predictor.* Bioinformatics, 2010. **26**(16): p. 2069-70.

76.   GTEx Consortium, *Human genomics. The Genotype-Tissue Expression (GTEx) pilot analysis: multitissue gene regulation in humans.* Science, 2015. **348**(6235): p. 648-60.

77.   Mele, M., et al., *Human genomics. The human transcriptome across tissues and individuals.* Science, 2015. **348**(6235): p. 660-5.

78.   Quinlan, A.R. and I.M. Hall, *BEDTools: a flexible suite of utilities for comparing genomic features.* Bioinformatics, 2010. **26**(6): p. 841-842.

79.   Li, H. and R. Durbin, *Fast and accurate short read alignment with Burrows-Wheeler transform.* Bioinformatics, 2009. **25**(14): p. 1754-60.

80.   Pickrell, J.K., et al., *Understanding mechanisms underlying human gene expression variation with RNA sequencing.* 2010. **464**: p. 768.

81.   Skelly, D.A., et al., *A powerful and flexible statistical framework for testing hypotheses of allele-specific gene expression from RNA-seq data.* Genome Research, 2011. **21**(10): p. 1728-1737.

82.   Gelman, A.C., John B.; Stern, Hal S.; Rubin, Donald B., *Bayesian Data Analysis*. 2nd ed. ed. Texts in Statistical Science. 2004: Chapman & Hall/CRC.

83.   Gelman, A., *Prior distributions for variance parameters in hierarchical models (comment on article by Browne and Draper)*. Bayesian Anal., 2006. **1**(3): p. 515-534.

84.   Miller, J.A., et al., *Transcriptional landscape of the prenatal human brain*. Nature, 2014. **508**(7495): p. 199-206.

85.   Fombonne, E., *Epidemiology of Pervasive Developmental Disorders*. Pediatric Research, 2009. **65**: p. 591-598.

86.   Robinson, E.B., et al., *Examining and interpreting the female protective effect against autistic behavior*. Proceedings of the National Academy of Sciences, 2013. **110**(13): p. 5258-5262.

87.   Zerbino, D.R., et al., *Ensembl 2018*. Nucleic Acids Research, 2017. **46**(D1): p. D754-D761.

88.   Zhao, X., et al., *A unified genetic theory for sporadic and inherited autism*. Proc Natl Acad Sci U S A, 2007. **104**(31): p. 12831-6.

89.   Keren, H., G. Lev-Maor, and G. Ast, *Alternative splicing and evolution: diversification, exon definition and function*. Nat Rev Genet, 2010. **11**(5): p. 345-55.

90.   Yang, X., et al., *Widespread expansion of protein interaction capabilities by alternative splicing*. Cell, 2016. **164**(4): p. 805-817.

91.   El-Gebali, S., et al., *The Pfam protein families database in 2019*. Nucleic Acids Research, 2018. **47**(D1): p. D427-D432.

92.   Djebali, S., et al., *Landscape of transcription in human cells*. Nature, 2012. **489**(7414): p. 101-108.

93.   Rodriguez, J.M., et al., *APPRIS: annotation of principal and alternative splice isoforms*. Nucleic Acids Research, 2013. **41**(D1): p. D110-D117.

94.   Davydov, E.V., et al., *Identifying a High Fraction of the Human Genome to be under Selective Constraint Using GERP++*. PLOS Computational Biology, 2010. **6**(12): p. e1001025.

95.   Pollard, K.S., et al., *Detection of nonneutral substitution rates on mammalian phylogenies*. Genome Research, 2010. **20**(1): p. 110-21.

96.   Siepel, A., et al., *Evolutionarily conserved elements in vertebrate, insect, worm, and yeast genomes.* Genome Research, 2005. **15**(8): p. 1034-1050.

97.   Buja, A., et al., *Damaging Mutations are Associated with Diminished Motor Skills and IQ in Children on the Autism Spectrum.* bioRxiv, 2017.

98.   Smedley, D., et al., *The BioMart community portal: an innovative alternative to large, centralized data repositories.* Nucleic Acids Research, 2015. **43**(W1): p. W589-W598.

99.   Weyn-Vanhentenryck, S.M., et al., *Precise temporal regulation of alternative splicing during neural development.* Nature Communications, 2018. **9**(1): p. 2189.

100.   Iossifov, I., et al., *Low load for disruptive mutations in autism genes and their biased transmission.* Proceedings of the National Academy of Sciences, 2015. **112**(41): p. E5600.

101.   Doyle, J.P., et al., *Application of a translational profiling approach for the comparative analysis of CNS cell types.* Cell, 2008. **135**(4): p. 749-62.

102.   Heiman, M., et al., *A translational profiling approach for the molecular characterization of CNS cell types.* Cell, 2008. **135**(4): p. 738-48.

103.   Skene, N.G. and S.G.N. Grant, *Identification of Vulnerable Cell Types in Major Brain Disorders Using Single Cell Transcriptomes and Expression Weighted Cell Type Enrichment.* Frontiers in Neuroscience, 2016. **10**: p. 16.

104.   Finucane, H.K., et al., *Heritability enrichment of specifically expressed genes identifies disease-relevant tissues and cell types.* Nature Genetics, 2018. **50**(4): p. 621-629.

105.   Saunders, A., et al., *A Single-Cell Atlas of Cell Types, States, and Other Transcriptional Patterns from Nine Regions of the Adult Mouse Brain.* bioRxiv, 2018: p. 299081.

106.   Zeisel, A., et al., *Molecular Architecture of the Mouse Nervous System.* Cell, 2018. **174**(4): p. 999-1014.e22.

107.   Saunders, A., et al., *Molecular Diversity and Specializations among the Cells of the Adult Mouse Brain.* Cell, 2018. **174**(4): p. 1015-1030.e16.

108.   NCBI Resource Coordinators, *Database Resources of the National Center for Biotechnology Information.* Nucleic Acids Research, 2017. **45**(D1): p. D12-d17.

109.   Helsmoortel, C., et al., *A SWI/SNF-related autism syndrome caused by de novo mutations in ADNP.* Nature Genetics, 2014. **46**(4): p. 380-384.

110.   Ben-Shalom, R., et al., *Opposing Effects on NaV1.2 Function Underlie Differences Between SCN2A Variants Observed in Individuals With Autism Spectrum Disorder or Infantile Seizures.* Biological Psychiatry, 2017. **82**(3): p. 224-232.

111.   Keren, L., et al., *Massively Parallel Interrogation of the Effects of Gene Expression Levels on Fitness.* Cell, 2016. **166**(5): p. 1282-1294.e18.

112.   Gandal, M.J., et al., *The road to precision psychiatry: translating genetics into disease mechanisms.* Nature Neuroscience, 2016. **19**(11): p. 1397-1407.

113.   Qureshi, A.Y., et al., *Opposing brain differences in 16p11. 2 deletion and duplication carriers.* The Journal of Neuroscience, 2014. **34**(34): p. 11199-11211.

114.   Hanson, E., et al., *The cognitive and behavioral phenotype of the 16p11.2 deletion in a clinically ascertained population.* Biological Psychiatry, 2015. **77**(9): p. 785-93.

115.   D'Angelo, D., et al., *Defining the Effect of the 16p11.2 Duplication on Cognition, Behavior, and Medical Comorbidities.* JAMA Psychiatry, 2016. **73**(1): p. 20-30.

116.   Collins, F.S. and H. Varmus, *A New Initiative on Precision Medicine.* New England Journal of Medicine, 2015. **372**(9): p. 793-795.

117.   Geschwind, D.H. and M.W. State, *Gene hunting in autism spectrum disorder: on the path to precision medicine.* The Lancet Neurology, 2015. **14**(11): p. 1109-1120.

118.   Guy, J., et al., *Reversal of Neurological Defects in a Mouse Model of Rett Syndrome.* Science, 2007. **315**(5815): p. 1143-1147.

119.   Mei, Y., et al., *Adult restoration of Shank3 expression rescues selective autistic-like phenotypes.* Nature, 2016. **530**(7591): p. 481-484.

120.   Ehninger, D., et al., *Reversal of learning deficits in a Tsc2+/− mouse model of tuberous sclerosis.* Nature Medicine, 2008. **14**(8): p. 843-848.

121.   Matharu, N., et al., *CRISPR-mediated activation of a promoter or enhancer rescues obesity caused by haploinsufficiency.* Science, 2019. **363**(6424): p. eaau0629.